Being with the Body in Depth Psychology

W0091347

Featuring a foreword by Donald Kalsched, this important book examines the integration of the subjectively experienced body in the practice of depth psychology.

Barbara Holifield draws from philosophical perspectives, neuroscientific and infant research, developmental theory, and trauma studies to offer a comprehensive overview of embodiment within a relationally based psychoanalytic approach. Clinical vignettes demonstrate the critical value of working with the bodily-felt dimension of implicit relational memory and emphasize how bodily-felt sense facilitates access to feelings. The mythopoetic reality revealed in depth psychotherapeutic process weaves all of this into a tapestry of personal meaning. Here the body serves as a portal to the numinous—healing that goes far beyond the relief of symptoms to a renewed sense of aliveness.

This book offers guiding principles for psychotherapists and clinicians of all levels to engage the bodily basis of experience in their clinical practice. It will appeal to general readers interested in integrating mind and body, including those in the healing arts, fine arts, dance, athletics, meditation, yoga, and martial arts.

Barbara Holifield is a training analyst member of the C. G. Jung Institute of San Francisco. With decades of experience with somatic psychology, including the psychophysical work with trauma known as Somatic Experiencing, she has synthesized somatic work into a relationally based psychoanalytic approach. A deep feeling for the body pulses through her work. Barbara taught somatic psychology to graduate students at the California Institute of Integral Studies for over twenty years and continues to facilitate Authentic Movement internationally. Barbara is the author of several articles that explore embodiment, trauma, and our participation in the dream of the earth.

Being with the Body in Depth Psychology

Development, Trauma, and Transformation in the Unspoken Realm

Barbara Holifield

With a Foreword by Donald Kalsched

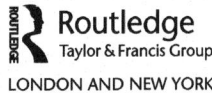

Routledge
Taylor & Francis Group

LONDON AND NEW YORK

Designed cover image: Rosalyn Driscoll, *Second Skin,* 2003–5, Steel, mixed media, 78" x 38" x 38". Photography by David Stansbury.

First published 2025
by Routledge
4 Park Square, Milton Park, Abingdon, Oxon OX14 4RN

and by Routledge
605 Third Avenue, New York, NY 10158

Routledge is an imprint of the Taylor & Francis Group, an informa business

British Library Cataloguing-in-Publication Data
A catalogue record for this book is available from the British Library

Library of Congress Cataloging-in-Publication Data
Names: Holifield, Barbara, author.
Title: Being with the body in depth psychology : development, trauma, and transformation in the unspoken realm / Barbara Holifield ; with a foreword by Donald Kalsched.
Description: Abingdon, Oxon ; New York, NY : Routledge, 2025. | Includes bibliographical references and index. |
Identifiers: LCCN 2024028098 (print) | LCCN 2024028099 (ebook) | ISBN 9781032286082 (paperback) | ISBN 9781032305905 (hardback) | ISBN 9781003305804 (ebook)
Subjects: MESH: Jungian Theory | Psychoanalytic Therapy—methods | Imagination | Movement—physiology | Psychophysiology
Classification: LCC RC506 .H64 2025 (print) | LCC RC506 (ebook) | NLM WM 460.5.J9 | DDC 616.89/17—dc23/eng/20240703
LC record available at https://lccn.loc.gov/2024028098
LC ebook record available at https://lccn.loc.gov/2024028099

ISBN: 978-1-032-30590-5 (hbk)
ISBN: 978-1-032-28608-2 (pbk)
ISBN: 978-1-003-30580-4 (ebk)

DOI: 10.4324/9781003305804

Typeset in Times New Roman
by codeMantra

This book is dedicated
to Don, his generosity, and his vision, and to
Tano, whose integrity is uniquely rooted in the mystery
of the non-conceptual

Contents

Acknowledgments

I owe a great deal to many. Whether one is a practitioner, a patient, or a student, engaging the depths of the embodied psyche is premised on relationships through which growth happens. This book arises from those kinds of relationships with others. I am profoundly grateful to those with whom I work, both students and patients. I am deeply moved by my analysands' courage to engage the depths of their inner world and to trust in me to accompany them in their analytic process. I am also profoundly moved by my students' courage to be with their own depths, enabling them to work with others consciously. I offer special acknowledgment to those patients and students who gave permission for me to use material from their work. All clinical descriptions are based on actual cases or composites of clinical casework. All identifying details and other elements have been disguised to protect the individuals' identities and preserve confidentiality.

I could not have written this book were it not for my husband, Don. Our rich and multithreaded conversations nourished my writing; his readings served as witness, inspiration, and counterpoint.

I bow with gratitude to the land where I dwell, Mount Tamalpais, and its more-than-human inhabitants. The natural world forever opens me to the vast sensorial realm. It sustains and guides me.

I bow to my particular body, which offers me rather potent doses of ecstasy and misery in, fortunately, unequal measure. This keeps me "awake," humble, grateful, and in a lifelong process of weaving awareness of myself with myself, all of which, thankfully, allows me to thrive well enough.

Acknowledgment must go to the soul-sustaining intimacy of friends. Some contributed directly through conversations and reading sections of the book at just the right moments, as did Rosalyn Driscoll and Robin Greenberg. I am grateful to Robert Tyminski for his 2024 translation of Rilke's *Sonnets to Orpheus, part 2, number 1*. Others contributed indirectly through love, encouragement, and support. I have deep gratitude for my Authentic Movement peer group of 30 years, without whom I would not be who I am.

My windows of perception of the utter entwinement of body and psyche blew open wide in undergraduate studies with Alton Wasson. I am forever grateful for his recognition of and faith in me. Edward Maupin's vision of the embodied psyche and his welcome to me as his apprentice set me on a deeply personal and professional path.

In the late 1980s, I found professional support for my interest in the significance of the body in Jungian Analysis at the "Professional Enrichment Program in Jungian Theory and Practice," where I first studied with Don Kalsched and Robin van Loben Sels. Their continued brilliant pursuit of that which wants and needs to be known has been a source of inspiration.

I am indebted to the C. G. Jung Institute of San Francisco for its soulful professional support—including the profoundly personal support of my analyst and consultants. I found the institutional openness there that I needed to pursue my calling. Joan Chodorow's pioneering work with the "moving imagination" has played an essential role.

The late Janet Adler's unwavering dedication to listening to what the body knows—in movement and stillness, emotionally and spiritually—and to practice this in community gave me a home to know what I know. My years of study with her were invaluable.

I am deeply grateful to Ursula Wirtz, who generously contributed to this book's coming to be through her thorough reading, enthusiasm, honest critique, and kind spirit. I additionally want to acknowledge the Analyst and Activism group spearheaded by Andrew Samuels. His support of Jungians widening and deepening the field through political action and publication, including this book, impacts many. Through my participation in that group, I met Ursula and developed great admiration for her courageous work, particularly with women who have been traumatized by war and political violence. Women's bodies are often the target of that unspeakable violence. I honor her courage to engage at this collective level of horror and suffering while maintaining ground in love and possibility.

I am indebted to Joel Ruimy for his steady, kind presence and eye for what I was up to in my writing. His careful copyediting brought clarity to the book. I am grateful to Suzi Naiburg for her invaluable insights and guidance on writing.

Chapter 7 is partly derived from my article, "Trauma, Soul, and the Body in Jungian Analysis," published in *Jung Journal: Culture and Psyche* and copyright 2020, by the Taylor & Francis Group. It is used with permission of Taylor & Francis, and with acknowledgment to the C. G. Jung Institute of San Francisco, publishers of the *Jung Journal*. I am also grateful to Linda Hogan for permission to use her poem *The Way In*, published in 2008 by CoffeeHouse Press and used with their permission. I acknowledge the Museum of Osteopathic Medicine for permission to reprint their image of an intact nervous system from the brain downward. Special thanks go to Rosalyn Driscoll, who gave permission to use images of her sculpture *Second Skin*.

Foreword

Donald Kalsched

Backstory

I have known Barbara Holifield for 40 years and have followed with great interest her developing ideas about the question: "How do we heal the psychological wounds left by early childhood trauma?" Like all intrepid explorers, she has not been content to accept the prevailing assumptions of Jungian psychology or psychoanalytic thought in general, but has always been called "over the horizon" of the known and accepted theories to explore "new lands"—many of them still uncharted by mainstream analytic thought. Always a seeker, she has had a passion for "unconventional" healing methods, especially those involving the body and the immediacy of *emotional experience in the body*. And she has not been afraid to sail into areas where the existing maps say only "Beware! Here there be dragons!" Finally, after a lifetime of exploring, writing, and developing her ideas—and now as a well-respected Jungian analyst—she has decided to present her own unique synthesis. This book is the result.

The core of this book is the author's work with early-trauma survivors who have been driven out of their inner worlds, and out of their feeling-bodies, into an external frame of reference and a *pathological accommodation* (Brandchaft, 2007) with the concrete literalisms of a polarized and polarizing world. These are people whose very vitality and emotional aliveness has been stolen from them by a sophisticated *system of defenses*, designed to save and protect them from further trauma—but ultimately stranding them in an emotional desert, cut off from their childhood vulnerabilities and from their deep heart's core. These heroic survivors of childhood trauma have learned to play all the notes written for them by the outer world, but the music is gone, and they don't know how to get it back.

Holifield's book is about finding a way back to that music—the forgotten music of a spontaneous, expressive, fully lived life. And for her, the "way in" is through the body, where all the feelings, sensations, and scraps of unformulated experience from early life lie dormant as "implicit processes" waiting to be awakened and led back across the threshold of dissociation into relationship and into a renewed experience of aliveness. But how to access the hidden resources of the body—and how to integrate these resources with the mythopoetic and symbolic understandings of conventional Jungian theory and practice? That is the task the author sets for herself, and the result is what I believe to be an important contribution to our understanding, and to the field of depth psychology in general.

Our Collaboration

I am especially pleased to offer this Foreword to her book because of the collaborative and synergistic nature of our relationship over many years. As an active and creative participant in an educational program I initiated back in the 1980s called the "Professional Enrichment Program in Jungian Theory and Practice," Barbara has both tracked the evolution of my own "neo-Jungian" ideas on trauma, and contributed to shaping them with her body-sensitive methods and commitments.

While my emphasis has been on the structure and dynamics of a defensive *structural system* that I began to see in early-trauma patients' dream-material (a dissociative system I called the "Self-care system"), and while I was concerned in a major way with theoretical links between Object-relations theory and Jung's psychology, Barbara was already breaking new ground in the area of HOW to work with such patients, and HOW to bypass the formidable defensive forces impacting their lives, in order to enhance the healing process. Now, 40 years later, our personal explorations and discoveries have evolved and matured independently, and so the links and connections between our respective contributions are all the more compelling and exciting.

In a Plenary lecture at the Congress of the International Association for Analytical Psychology in Vienna in 2019, I moved my own thinking forward onto "new ground" by focusing on the crucial importance of affect, feelings, and the immediacy of experience in the body, in our work with early-childhood-trauma survivors. I made the statement that many of our patients have "had their hearts broken before they had hearts to break." Although I didn't know it then, I was describing patients whose fundamental experience-worlds were left fragmented and unformulated (Stern, 1997), and for whom severe, systemic dissociation was necessary for their self-regulation. This was a level of dissociation deeper and more profound than what Jung usually described in his work with "complexes."

At this developmentally earlier and more severe level, dissociative defenses were working to maintain the fragments of atomized unformulated experience in their dis-aggregated state, i.e., to prevent them from formulating into the "molecules" of affect-images and other imaginative content that could be used for symbolic processing, dreaming, imagining, and reflecting.[1] The reason for this was the amount of fear and anxiety in these patients' inner worlds. So if you asked these patients "what they were feeling" they couldn't tell you. It was still all a blur. Their experience hadn't "formulated" yet, and remained in fragments lodged in the "somatic unconscious." Jung was one of the first to teach us that primitive affects are not yet feelings, and are not yet accessible through the usual verbal/interpretive approach of psychoanalysis. We are slowly learning how to gain access to this material, and Barbara's descriptions of "body-based inquiries" in Chapter 3 of her book provide many useful ways of working more directly with immediate experience in the body. I have personally found that many of her suggestions make emotion and feelings more accessible, and thereby deepen my process with patients.

In my own early work with trauma survivors, I discovered that my patients' well-meaning efforts to get in touch with their feelings were hijacked by self-critical or reality-denying defensive "thoughts" that would take them immediately out of their bodies and into their heads. A careful examination of their dreams revealed an inner "fifth column" of powerful personified "beings" ostensibly designed to undermine any feelings of vulnerability or openness, leading them away from their own psychic pain or innocent childhood dependency. I realized that I was witnessing *an archetypal system of dissociative defenses* in action. The system operated like auto-immune disease in the body. Healthy affect-precursors or new life-full energies (seeking to formulate and become conscious) were mistaken (by the system) for dangerous intrusion and either violently attacked or seduced into reality-denying "spiritualized" illusions or "mentalized" obsessions. Violent demons collaborated with spell-casting, over-protective "guardian angels"[2] to prevent feelings from emerging—to "kill" or encapsulate them. Trauma, I had learned, is an "injury to the capacity to feel" (Russell, 1999), and the systemic dissociation I was witnessing in these patients' dreams was how this injury happened.

As I became better acquainted with the Self-care system, I realized that the *raison d'être* of the whole structure was to preserve and protect the imperishable personal spirit or soul of the patient by making sure this core of innocence did not enter experience too soon or without proper mediation. This core of vulnerability and aliveness was protected or persecuted "by the angels." Meanwhile, the empirical wounded child within who carried all the wounds and pain of early trauma was not allowed to enter feeling-life in the human world. He/she was protected (as good) or persecuted and shamed (as bad) but never allowed *into relationship* where the "good" and the "bad" could be rendered into a negotiated "democracy of the psyche" and the extreme splitting of early trauma could be healed. This humanization of the archetypal system can only happen in relationship, and Holifield's new book is intensely relational.

I've given this brief review of the Self-care system because, to my great pleasure, it has become one of several useful maps in the author's somatically informed psychotherapy practice, and she uses it regularly in her work. This is especially clear in Chapters 4 and 7 of the book, where there are extensive case write-ups illustrating how the *wounded child*, protected by the Self-care system, comes into view symbolically after dissociative defenses have been identified and softened through the author's particular way of attending to the felt-sensations "underneath" the patient's conscious awareness of what is transpiring inwardly. The inner "child" then becomes a further "way in" to un-remembered traumatic pain and eventually to healing.

In this and other ways, the author illustrates how the mythopoetic psyche contributes—through dreams, imagination, and artwork—to the more experiential work with the body, bringing in "dual vectors" of experience that deepen the work and contribute a dimension of *meaning* that eludes us if we work within only one vector or the other. By attending to dreams and to the feelings surrounding the inner child, the inter-psychic field of the transference is amplified by the intra-psychic wisdom of the psyche's mythic depths. Kairos intersects Chronos, and the Numinous may appear. I will expand on this briefly below.

But first, I would like to note some of the fundamental *orienting assumptions* and emphases of Holifield's work in general, illuminated throughout the book and especially in the context of her case studies. These assumptions are now becoming mainstream in the treatment of early trauma and dissociation, but it has taken many years for the field to catch up to them.

Foundational Assumptions of the Book

- *Experience over Explanations:* The author notes that the body is a direct source of knowledge and the ground of affective life in general—if we know how to attend it. Such attention shifts the emphasis of meaning-making away from language and symbolization to immediate experience. For example, noticing the breath and the "felt sense" of moment-to-moment bodily sensations provide access to the "deep body," also known as *the interoceptive system*. This pre-reflective, pre-verbal system is well below the threshold of consciousness and Damasio (2021) posits it as the very origin of consciousness and subjectivity. It is comprised of our deep viscera in communication with the autonomic and sympathetic nervous system. It is where a felt sense of aliveness resides, where self-regulation occurs, and where unformulated experience begins to formulate as subjective awareness. Hence, if we want to heal trauma *at the root of its manifestation*, we will have to become acquainted with this deep psychophysiological level, and resist our tendency to cognitively override the body. Holifield notes that there is an abundance of thoughtful literature *about the body*, but much less describing the body *as experienced*. Her book is an effort to help fill this gap.
- *Relationship Is Primary:* Infant research supports the fact that the body is intrinsic to relational life, and that infants have the capacity for primary intersubjectivity at the very beginning of life. It is in and through the body that relationship begins. Disruptions in one's earliest relationship with the primary caregiver are synonymous with disruption of the integral unity of psyche and body, and the inevitable beginning of dissociative defenses. What was injured relationally must be repaired relationally. Therefore, intimate attention to the moment-to-moment inwardly experienced body-based sensations of *both* the analyst and analysand becomes a crucial "field" of relational awareness in a somatically sensitive depth psychotherapy. Patient and analyst move through a patient's most troubling wounds and vulnerabilities through what the Boston Change Process Study Group (Bruschweiler-Stern et al., 2018) calls "body-based inter-affectivity." Hurts that lie in the nether lands of the body's

early unformulated experience remain isolated unless the therapeutic relationship is open to the un-thinkable, to the un-feelable—to the most "primitive" language of the body—as experience begins to formulate.

- *The Sensorial Basis of Emotion:* Emotions become known through sensations in the deep body first. The profundity of sensory awareness is a bridge to conscious affective life. Attending to the breath and to felt-sensations in the body as well as to spontaneous gestures, postures, or involuntary movements often leads to direct experience of emotions. Because much of our earliest traumatic experience is unformulated and remains so because of dissociative defenses, exploration of emotional life must begin with the body's sensations, and must proceed through micro-attention to the moment-by-moment evolution of experience. For example, dropping down (with a guide) into the sensing body—each sensorial, kinesthetic, imagistic, or affective nook and cranny of it—then noticing what happens, and what happens next, such as tightening or loosening, surging or retreating, pulsing or quiet stillness—these ways of attending open up the basic building blocks of affective experience and eventually, through further co-regulation, to more differentiated feelings. This process is equivalent to a slow building-up of what Paul Russell (1999, pp. 45–46) would call "affect-competency." And the movement is always "from the bottom up."
- *Necessity of the Therapist's Own Body-awareness:* In the many case examples and vignettes throughout the book, the author describes how powerful unconscious psycho-physical forces are constellated in the countertransference while working with early-trauma survivors. The clinician's awareness of his/her own bodily states can be key in the transformative unfolding of the patient's affect-life, and in attending—and ultimately resolving—the frequent *enactments* that occur as unformulated experience reaches the threshold of consciousness through repetition in the analytic partnership.
- *The Poetics of Embodiment in Groups:* The author devotes all of Chapter 9 to how affective life and what she calls "interaffectivity" come alive in Authentic Movement groups. Based upon many years of participating in, and then teaching, this method, she vividly describes how the body as experienced in stillness and movement becomes the medium of non-verbal, sensate exploration, slowly evolving into carefully structured periods of verbal dialogue. The result, she reports is a highly attuned intersubjective field in which participants find the emotional safety and attunement that allows emotional transformation often not found in dyadic, verbal forms of therapy. I personally have experienced these groups and can testify to their power and healing potential.
- *Wider Cultural and Spiritual Implications:* The author convincingly states that her somatically informed depth psychotherapeutic approach has wider implications than just the healing of dissociation in the consulting room. Based on years of experience with these methods, she believes that the transformational processes set in motion by inwardly focused attention to the body in the presence of a compassionate other, provide a deep sense of aliveness beyond the polarized

extremes of defenses in general, and that this often opens to a sublime sense of wonder, cultivating the lost—and now found—

- "dimensional life that one longs for." What she refers to as "the body's deep ontological understanding of Being," when touched, can lead to a profound experience of the numinous and to realities that lie "beyond" our usual embeddedness in a one-dimensional world. With increased access to both feelings and the imaginal world comes a renewed sense of soulful aliveness and meaning.

Identifying the Self-care System through the Body and the Imagination

Chapters 4 and 7 in the book contain case vignettes that illustrate how the author works sensitively back and forth between a highly experiential body-sensitive approach on the one hand, and an imaginal sensitivity on the other. The result is a special awareness of the wounded "child" in both herself and her patient—an inner part of their shared selves, their "embodied inter-affectivity" that emerges from deep unconscious communication between them.

For example, the terror and panic of her patient "Lucinda" about a threatened abandonment by her partner stimulated in Barbara some "middle-of-the-night rememberings" in her own body of herself as a little girl alone, haunted by some un-namable terror, frozen in fear and too terrified to call out. These deep "syntonic" countertransference responses, mediated by the unconscious "field," led to the author's increased sensitivity to the terrified "little girl" in the patient. As she and her patient attended the dissociated (hence necessarily imagined) feelings of this "little girl," scraps of memories emerged in the patient, and she began to cry from this very young, un-sharable deep place in herself.

The "little girl" previously frozen in fear was suddenly and movingly in tears. Then, with her therapist's help, the patient was able to imagine her adult self comforting the little girl, holding her on her lap and against her chest. This relational moment and many that followed led to a deeper capacity in the patient to open outwardly into a trusting reliance on her analyst and inwardly to a "deep feeling of peace" inside.

One of the places where the author's expertise in working with the body has expanded my own understanding of how the Self-care system manifests in clinical process is the discovery that *there is often a bodily basis for the defensive structures that I have identified as the Self-care system.* Knowing this, and sensitizing the patient to the bodily form taken by the "Dis-inspired false-narrative" delivered by dissociative defenses into the treatment situation, can help the patient "see" how the defense operates and help in the process of dis-identification from its intractable and "addictive" powers. For example, often the self-protective mechanisms of the "system" manifest in the patient's postural expression—a pattern of tightening in the shoulders or clenching the jaw, repetitive tense movements in the legs, restricted breathing—can all, when sensed within a safe and compassionate field, lead to purposefully releasing the tensional patterns giving rise to greater understanding of their unconscious operation as survival strategies.

In the past, my tendency has been to see how the defenses move the patient "into the head" or "into the left hemisphere" or "into a pathological 'mind-psyche'." But it is clear from Barbara's book that archetypal defenses are not just mentalizing defenses or "head trips," although they frequently start out that way.

Another case ("Eva") in Chapter 7 illustrates some of the complexities of working with the inner child as it begins to emerge from the protection of the Self-care system. The patient often painted images from her imagination, and frequently out-pictured a lost child in her artwork. Reflecting on this image, she was finally able to "confess" that the little girl was a part of herself and that it contained all the "bad" feelings she suffered from her shaming mother. The patient was convinced that this child contained the "truth" about herself. Hence, in compliance with her defensive "system," she had made a pact with herself never to need anything— never to upset anyone, never to cry. In other words, as the author observes, this was the child who fell into the grips of her violent dark angel, becoming convinced she was "bad" and colluding with the dark angel's conviction of her badness. The continual corrosive inner messages from this part of the Self-care system, concretized and reinforced her shame-ridden identification.

Consequently, in the transference, the patient continually strove to be "good" so that her therapist wouldn't be angry with her or abandon her. This amounted to a retreat into the arms of the bright angel and an unconscious insistence that her therapist play this inflated role, while she maintained her "goodness" as an equally inflated, perpetually "innocent" child. As the author trenchantly notes, psychological integration of the good and bad was not possible for her patient, trapped in this situation, and so the therapeutic process soon bogged down.

Such impasses are by now legendary in the field of our work with trauma and severe dissociation. Donnel Stern (2010, p. 189) has noted that, because such impasses are so early and so embedded in relational failures of the child's earliest environment, any healing of dissociation must therefore also come *through relationship* and that the way this happens is through *enactments*. In the messy process of an enactment, unformulated experience reaches the surface in the form of an emotional crisis—a crisis now delivered into the treatment situation. And this, says Stern, is the only way for unformulated experience to become conscious. One cannot, says Stern, "interpret" one's way out of such impasses. One has to relive them—repeat them—hopefully to a different outcome.

Barbara Holifield then gives a beautiful description of her own enactment—how she and her patient suffered through it, and how ultimately, by surviving their mutual anger and disillusionment with each other, they each became more real and more genuinely intimate with, and open to, each other. In other words, the real, empirical inner child (of both therapist and patient) finally makes her appearance in the field, and brings with her all the tenderness and vulnerability that were a part of early unbearable suffering.

Finally, and with remarkable perceptiveness, the author describes this as a process through which the bright and dark angels in the Self-care system—inflated powers with which the patient was alternatively identified—are humanized through the *sturm und drang* of the enactment itself. This is a step beyond the polarization of defenses and the polarization of the world.

Her book represents the very best of current psychoanalytic writing. In an increasingly dehumanizing world, it contributes to the humanizing of us all.

Topsham, Maine
March 2024

Notes

1 Many years ago, Wilfred Bion described such fragmented "inchoate elements" as "Beta-elements" developmentally prior to later, more mature symbol-producing "Alpha-function." See "A Theory of Thinking" in Bion, W. (1967), *Second Thoughts* (pp. 100–120).

2 I frequently use a painting by Willian Blake, *The Good and Evil Angels Fight for Possession of a Child*, to illustrate how the Self-care system "works." In the image, a "Dark Angel" and a "Bright Angel" each protect and/or persecute a good/bad child in their tyrannical care. The "child" is simultaneously both innocent and corrupted; angelically "good" and demonically "bad" (depending upon which angel possesses him) but never both (humanization of archetypes, i.e., incarnation). See Kalsched (2013), *Trauma and the Soul*, Routledge.

References

Brandchaft, B. (2007). Systems of pathological accommodation and change in analysis. *Psychoanalytic Psychology 24*, 667–687.

Bruschweiler-Stern, N., Lyons-Ruth, K., Morgan, A. C., Nahum, J. P., & Reis, B. (2018). Moving through and being moved by: Embodiment in development and in the therapeutic relationship. *Psychoanalytic Inquiry, 38*(5), 311–326.

Damasio, A. (2021). *Feeling and Knowing: Making Minds Conscious*. New York: Pantheon Books.

Russell, P. (1999). *Trauma, Repetition and Affect Regulation*, J. G. Teicholz & D. Kriegman (Eds.). New York: Rebus Press.

Stern, D. B. (1997). *Unformulated Experience: From Dissociation to Imagination in Psychoanalysis*. Hillsdale, NJ: The Analytic Press.

——— (2010). *Partners in Thought: Working with Unformulated Experience, Dissociation, and Enactment*. New York, London: Routledge.

Introduction

But where the danger is, also grows the saving power.

(Friedrich Hölderlin, 2014)

As I embarked on this writing endeavor, many memories and callings arose. My early life was saturated with developmental trauma. What plagued my family then is still all too common today in this culture: Unresolved grief and trauma leading to addiction, acts of desperation resulting in destructive behaviors, suicide, and premature death. At a very young age, however, some part of myself foresaw a different trajectory.

I was four or five years old when I dreamt my family was in a space rocket that crashed on another planet. Everyone was killed but me. By mid-life, this was so: My parents, three siblings, and two brothers-in-law were all dead. Recent research assessing adverse childhood experiences predicts emotional difficulties in later life, along with illness and shortened life expectancy (Giano, Wheeler & Hubach, 2020). A great deal of my experience growing up was horrific. Sadly, this is true for untold numbers in the United States and elsewhere (Briggs et al., 2021). This undercurrent of pain pulses through our populace and likely plays a large part in feeding the divisiveness and othering so rampantly spreading throughout the world. My need to live in an alternate reality rather than the one I was born into was a blessing that silently drew me downward and inward, toward soul. This pull seemed never to let me go; even when I turned my back on it, it never let me forget. For many years, fear was one of my most prevalent feeling states. However, rather than withdrawing, some inner courage pulled me forward, even when facing what terrified me the most.

This is also true of writing this book. This other, seemingly wiser part of me is what Jung called the Self, the archetypal energy that is the central organizing principle of the psyche. Jung recognized psyche's intrinsic thrust toward wholeness. Trauma can severely impede this dynamic of the psyche (Kalsched, 2013). My need to live in an alternate reality from the one I grew up in was, on the one hand, dissociative, protecting me from being overwhelmed by more pain than I could bear. Yet, paradoxically, once I was old enough to reflect on the dream, it helped me

DOI: 10.4324/9781003305804-1

to feel the depth of my sadness and make sense of the reality I felt I was living in—no one was "there"—and I, too, had "gone away" from my feelings. The dream simultaneously confirmed what I needed: to dwell in my own earthly body—to sense and feel—embracing this as part of the meaning of my life on this precious planet earth. My dream depicts the disruption of psyche indwelling soma—I left my body, my earth—when it felt to me that everyone else in my family had as well. Psyche indwelling soma can be either fortified or impaired in developmental life. Resilience, whether intrinsic or externally supported, can buffer such inner disruption.

I have been blessed with fine teachers along my way, which I am sure accounts for much of my resilience. In a tiny alternative Catholic high school in the Texas Panhandle, a religion teacher was genuinely interested in what I experienced as sacred. Literature and philosophy classes encouraged soulful inquiry, and its expression through poetry that embraced the true spectrum of our feelings. Rather than striving for perfect grades in all subjects, the school asked us to dedicate our energy to what interested us the most. I rode my spirited horse, which my grandfather had the foresight to get for me, across the vast open landscape of the great plains, witnessing countless sunsets that filled me with awe. The horse, which must have been sedated when we bought it for a low price at auction, was far from easy. Determined to sustain this relationship with wildness, I recognized her as my first Zen teacher, though I don't recall ever being introduced to Buddhism.

The guidance that I found, and that seemed to find me, is akin to that which orients a person toward what Jung referred to as individuation, the process of aligning with one's true nature. Jung describes it as a call to the spirit of the depths rather than the spirit of the times. He understood the second half of life to be that phase in which a call to soul was likely activated. However, for some, childhood trauma can impact the psyche in such a way that the crack between the worlds—the mundane (stripped of feeling, thus meaning) and the sacred—opens. Such a traumatized young person, like me, can find themselves adrift in the world many others occupy. Pulled into this other realm, I found my dream world offered an alternative perspective on life and, at times, hope and a rather uncanny source of guidance.

By the grace of something much larger than myself, I recognized that a traditional school was likely to amplify a pull toward dissociative behaviors. Instead, I chose an alternative—Prescott College. The foundation of the school's pedagogy was that learning be experiential, collaborative, and self-directed while incorporating in-depth study and breadth of knowledge. The primary classroom was the wilderness—the natural world. Only one or two subjects were studied at any time, so whether the course focused on dreams or environmental science, about a quarter to a half of it occurred in the field, typically in the wilderness. For example, if studying dreams, the first weeks were dedicated to reading, seminars, and experiential work with dreams. In the remaining weeks, we would journey as a small collective, hiking, rafting, or kayaking somewhere in the stunning wilds of the southwest. During this time, we worked in groups with our dreams and Jungian active imagination, exploring both the inner and outer landscape and the reciprocal affect of one upon the other. In this way, I was introduced to Jung, dreamwork, and the self-knowledge that arises from exploring symbols. In the context of a small community pursuing inquiry-based meaning, immersion in wilderness (inner and outer) was transformational. It clarified the path before me. You will see the centrality of our relationship to the natural world and its indissoluble bond with health woven throughout the case studies I will present in this book.

The effect of this approach to education was that it anchored the central source of knowing within. Though I would not have been able to articulate this at the time, it countered the driving intent of the dissociative defenses—to dismiss and disconnect one from core vulnerability—that were at work within. It kept me tethered to soul, as did companionship and the natural world. This was in the late 1970s, and the human potential movement was blossoming. I studied humanistic, Rogerian, and gestalt therapy, in which working with how inner dynamics live in the body was front and center. I was also introduced to modalities that would become core to the field of Somatics. Deeply affected by these, as part of my undergraduate degree, I designed an independent study program at Esalen Institute to further this current of learning.

While my soul was aligned to the sacred, and there was a sense of the deep rightness within, the insidious residue of shame rooted in early trauma continued to implode in my body. It was an immense work to hold this polarity that existed in me. I longed to be and move in the wilderness with strength and pleasure. I longed to relate to myself and others without a sense of shame that could sometimes drown out all joy. Early on, I knew I would study psychology because it offered some possibility that I longed for. I knew I had to understand what had happened in my family. I knew that working with dreams was my calling. Yet, I had to work in and through my body to do so.

Over time, through focused body-based work consciously grounded in psychological process, I discovered that the release of long-held patterns of dissociation and fear opened the door to an immediacy with life. This work unfolded in relationships through which I learned, in a cellular way, to receive rather than guard against being touched literally and metaphorically. Though it took many years, a time came in which I emerged from the mists and could enter a fuller state of presence.

From a clinical perspective, the mists I refer to can be seen as dissociated veils of unformulated experience. Throughout the book, I will discuss how unformulated experience is worked with as it arises in the therapeutic relationship and becomes symbolized in image and word. I emphasize cultivating the richness of direct bodily experience such that symbolization partakes in bodily-felt sense rather than arising *out* of it. In this way, symbols and words do not hold a hierarchical value over the body; instead, these remain intimately entwined.

By the time I entered Jungian analysis, a way of knowing through the body was intrinsically woven into my being. Though the analysts I had the honor to work with were not formally trained in attending to inner body-based processes, they were open to my experience, such that the transformational process incorporated the fullness of my otherwise fragmented self.

There was a particular moment as an undergraduate student when I knew that for me to practice psychotherapy, such an endeavor must include the body. My education had afforded me the opportunity to experience some of the pioneers of the field, including Charlotte Selver, Gabriella Roth, Stan Groff, Emily Conrad Da'oud, Anna Halprin, and Bonnie Bainbridge Cohen. I familiarized myself with Reich and studied Bioenergetics. Later, I dove into Arnie Mindell's Dreambody Work and Eugene Gendlin's Focusing. Perhaps because of the cellular depths of the tensional patterns I held and the need—though at the time unconscious—for direct touch, I was most affected by the work of the Rolf Method of Structural Integration. Upon completing my undergraduate degree, I apprenticed with the psychologist Edward Maupin, who oriented through a Jungian lens and had trained with Ida Rolf and Fritz Perls. At that time, we were part of a small community in San Diego. We developed a psychologically processed-based approach to hands-on myofascial bodywork, with attuned and noninvasive touch as the guiding principle. Out of this, the Institute for Psycho-Structural Balancing was founded. Later, I continued training and certification through the Rolf Institute and with the Upledger Institute for CranioSacral Therapy. I moved to New York City, where my practice became primarily focused on working with psychotherapists, many of whom were also exploring how to deepen somatic awareness in their work with others, whether they were Bioenergetic, Neo-Reichian, Core Energetic, Freudian, or Jungian psychoanalysts.

While I am certain that there are realms of psyche-soma that can only be contacted through direct touch, after a dozen years of practice, I decided to no longer do hands-on work with the body. Depth psychotherapeutic work that integrates the use of touch is extraordinarily profound but not appropriate for all. My shift away from hands-on work was based on this clinical reality and my personal individuation process.

My early mentor, Edward Maupin, had also studied with Mary Whitehouse, who pioneered the practice of Authentic Movement. This spoke to me in the deepest of ways. Through this approach, I truly learned to listen inwardly. I learned to move from a source rooted deep within and to be with the fertile ground of conscious stillness. I learned to trust that descent into the pain and darkness of the bodily-based psyche was a portal to transformation. I discovered beauty lived in and through me. I learned the extraordinary depths of our interconnectedness. The South African term *Umbutu*, meaning *I am because you are*, gets at this interconnected beauty, its reality, and its basis in love and relatedness. Since then, I have practiced and taught Authentic Movement, also known as Moving in Depth, and I've integrated it into my analytical work with individuals.

I have oriented my teaching practice of Authentic Movement, specifically toward professionals in the field of psychotherapy. I know of no better or more elegant practice for training psychotherapists to learn, through experience, the potency of body-based awareness in the use of self. I think of Moving in Depth for psychotherapists in parallel with meditation practice for those interested in cultivating acceptance and an inner witness to life's unfolding—the extraordinary range of the sacred, both immanent and transcendent. However, Movement in Depth is relational; thus, it shapes a relational form of meditation. Group and cross-cultural group practice yield particularly rich results in bringing consciousness to bear on the subtle ways we mutually influence each other and the healing potency that can emerge from this.

When I dedicated my work to Jungian Analysis, a feeling for the body pulsed deep within me and has remained integral to my practice. As I dove further into my studies in the late 1980s, I had the good fortune to meet Don Kalsched at the Professional Enrichment Program in Jungian Theory and Practice, where he was shaping an approach to working with trauma that recognized the significance of the body. Over the years, his work, its deep relational foundation, and dedication to understanding how psyche and soma can be disrupted have been enormously influential and supportive of my interests. In 2000, I began in-depth training with Peter Levine, working with the psychophysical manifestations of trauma, known as Somatic Experiencing. This work and the neuroscience that now illuminates the body–mind relationship are intrinsic to my practice.

This book explores the intricacies of working with the body as experienced in the course of depth psychotherapy. Jung speaks of psychology as being nothing if not experience (1966/1943). Many seeking psychotherapy, like myself, long for soul, perhaps even require a link to soul, or what they sense as sacred, to be explicitly part of a psychotherapeutic process. Jungian and post-Jungian work both do this. However, many are not drawn to Jung or depth psychology because it seems too conceptual. Focusing on embodiment and leaning into the felt sense of the reality of the psyche, the foundation of which is being with the *feeling* of feelings, grounds the work in what is essential in our time—the healing of personal and transgenerational trauma that otherwise threatens to undermine our ability to function as a people enduringly connected to the earth community. The focus of this book is not to replace what has come before but to highlight the bodily basis of psyche's unfolding process.

For those for whom the body is foreign territory, I hope to bring a feel for being in the body into a kind of immediacy of experience so that even if it is not where one is most drawn, at least one could find satisfaction in exploring the territory like one would relish walking the streets of a foreign country. While some have more proclivity toward the body, some toward thinking, feeling, or intuition, being with the body as experienced is not a matter of typology but is innate to us all. Our culture, training, development, and trauma influence our felt awareness of this.

Much of this book will focus on how psychological injury and trauma disrupts embodiment. Yet, as healing is set in motion, the body can be the portal for transforming those injuries.

A patient of mine, adept at identifying her emotions, once asked me, "If all emotions are embodied phenomena, why do I feel befuddled when you ask me where I feel them in my body?" This book is a long reflection on that question. It is a meditation on embodiment. It is about its disruption and cultivation. It will be explored from the perspective of what is given and what is nurtured. Cultivation of the felt awareness of embodiment is its central theme.

References

Briggs, E. C., Amaya-Jackson, L., Putnam, K. T., & Putnam, F. W. (2021). All adverse childhood experiences are not equal: The contribution of synergy to adverse childhood experience scores. *American Psychologist 76*(2), 243–252. https://doi.org/10.1037/amp0000768

Giano, Z., Wheeler, D. L., & Hubach, R. D. (2020). The frequencies and disparities of adverse childhood experiences in the U.S. *BMC Public Health 20*, 1327. https://doi.org/10.1186/s12889-020-09411-z

Hölderlin, F., in Mauch, C. (2014). "But where the danger lies, also grows the saving power": Reflections on exploitation and sustainability. *Perspectives* 2014(1), 129–135.

Jung, C. G. (1966/1943). On the psychology of the unconscious. In *Two Essays on Analytic Psychology: Vol. 7. Collected Works*. Princeton, NJ: Bollingen Foundation.

Kalsched, D. (2013). *Trauma and the soul: A psycho-spiritual approach to human development and its interruption*. New York: Routledge.

Chapter 1

The Way In

The Way In

Sometimes the way to milk and honey is through the body.
Sometimes the way in is a song.
But there are three ways in the world: dangerous, wounding,
and beauty.
To enter stone, be water.
To rise through hard earth, be plant
desiring sunlight, believing in water.
To enter fire, be dry.
To enter life, be food.

(Linda Hogan, 2008, *The Way In*)

Beauty

It is early morning. I am standing by a confluence of two streams. The water is cascading down the mountain, having been replenished by several days of rain. In the present drought-stricken California landscape, this is a remarkable moment. I gesture, lifting my hands. Almost immediately, my *intent to move* joins a *sense of being moved* as my palms turn upward, elbows slightly bent. The movement is slow. My palms lift, now hovering level with my heart. The space between my hands widens. My attention is drawn to that vulnerable place in the center of my palms. I feel a sense of receptivity there, and something enters: the rumbling rush of sound as the stream pours over and around rocks as it courses down the mountain, the forest now saturated in color. This fullness enters my palms as a tingling aliveness that softens a background dread of fire and the pervasive thirst that had spread over the land and entered my bones. A silence enters me right alongside the rushing water. I feel inwardly replenished, fuller, though I had not been aware of the tensional grip of depletion. Walking back down the hill, I pass others. Though usually few words are shared on the trail, this morning, each person is infused with wonder. One tells me she can *hear* the mountain drinking in the water. I am struck by this atypical comment. Her tone conveys the tender way she is moved by this moment, by the meeting between her and the natural world, and now between us.

DOI: 10.4324/9781003305804-2

Our encounter and a couple of others that occur as I hike back down the trail accentuates this effervescent feel of connection. The rain has brought relief from an imminent danger of fire in our community. Wonder and relief combine.

Sometimes the *Way In* Is through the Body

There are many ways in. My conscious movement had a powerful galvanizing effect on my state of consciousness. By conscious movement here, I mean that as I move, my awareness is on the sensations I feel in my *inner* body, such as my breath, my heart pumping from the climb, and a tingling excitation streaming through me. In addition, I am aware of the natural world as it meets my *outer* body; I hear the coursing sound of water, the sight of thirsty redwoods whose multilayered trunks are now made lush with nuances of color from the rain. I welcome the spicy fragrance of bay trees, the caress of wind on my cheeks, and the gentle downward pull of gravity from the soles of my feet up through the very core of my body. When the impulse arises to lift my hands, I follow it, moving slowly so as to not lose track of any of what I am sensing, but to let the experience of moving now be included. Then the moment comes in which I am no longer initiating the movement. Rather, I feel I am moved; the gesture emerges. In turn, experiencing the gesture, a quiet wonderment animates me from within.

My movement becomes a gateway into a deeper intimacy with myself and the more-than-human world. A homecoming. In the beginning, I become keenly aware of how my living, breathing bodily self is utterly interdependent with the air that I gratefully take in. With this awareness revivified, it becomes nonsensical to wonder if the air I breathe is part of the external world or already part of my organism—from a functional systems perspective, no distinction can be made between an inner self and the outer air (Fuchs, 2018, p. 128). Next, through this practice of remembering by means of connecting with a felt sense of myself as an integral whole within the environment, I regain recognition of my ecological subjectivity, or ecological sense of self (Bateson, 1972, cited in Fuchs, 2018). A sense of hope is replenished as my experience of self expands. Walking back down the hill, I become aware of a renewed sense of my capacity to carry the world's suffering. I no longer feel that it weighs me down such that I am unable to act. Rather, my bodily self literally feels lighter and more spacious inside. I have a whole-bodied, felt sense of being in connection with the natural world and the life that pulses through it with uncanny intelligence. In time, I realize how this experience has buffered me from the pessimism and futility that were hovering within. In my daily life, I find it challenging not to push away the complexly layered tender feelings of love and loss associated with the ecological crisis because they unfold alongside the utter exasperation I experience living in a society so polarized that it seems we cannot act in our own best interests. As my sense of self expands I am able to reorient to possibilities that otherwise become buried in a pervasive pallor of dystopia cast by the overwhelming weight of the terrible daily news.

This inner reorientation is characterized by a more flexible sense of myself. When overwhelmed by what feels terrible, sometimes without even being conscious of it, I shut down and rigidify—somewhere deep in my body, and with that, so too my thoughts and feelings. Almost without realizing it, my attention then narrows toward my own immediate world. My experience on the mountain re-sensitizes me. Now, I remember in my own body just how vulnerable I am, and I believe, we are to re-traumatization when caught in the sticky details of traumatic pain. Turning toward what is bearable, perhaps even beautiful, whether found in the outer world, within myself, or in my relationships, allows an inner softening, a *way in* to more of my self than the part that shuts down when faced with more than I can metabolize. I know well that for myself and those with whom I work, this more spacious sense of self made possible by bodily-based awareness serves us well in everyday life, not just when in the grip of trauma. What is key in this turn to the inwardly felt body is "presence."

Presence

The bare awareness of the receptive spaciousness of our body–mind defines "presence." Bringing purposeful awareness to multifaceted sensorial perception, as I describe experiencing in my morning walk, is one *way in* to an experience of the body—where *inner* and *outer* body meet—serving as a gateway to "presence."

Presence can also be described as a state of being, inhabiting a quality of time, of "Now" (Heidegger, 2008). It is a state that has been desired, explored, valued, and elevated as close to the divine in many cultures.[1] As the field of somatic psychology and practices of mindfulness have gained scientific substantiation through the research of neuroscience, the term "presence" has become widely used. As happens with many words once taken into the broader collective, it has been trivialized by careless usage, often with commercial intent. Like all archetypal states, once stripped of experience, it is just an image, frequently used but emptied of lived meaning. By reconnecting the term to lived experience, its significance can be renewed. To be "present" in the "now" is to enter an experience of time the ancient Greeks referred to as *Kairos*. Building on the psychological nuance of the bodily-based qualities of awake, alert, centered, and grounded, with affective attunement, extends "presence" to include an emotional acuity with self, others, and the world. Such states are fundamental for differentiated awareness required for true I–Thou relations. When looking through an intersubjective lens, the relational potential that can be activated in states of presence is made visible. When entered, whether with meditative intent or unexpectedly, fertile ground is laid for experiences of the numinous.

Being with the body in Depth Psychotherapy is a potent avenue for accessing affect. Cultivating presence furthers this, enriching felt experience of the myriad expression of vitality (Stern, 2010) inherent in affect. A resonant analogy is to attend to felt sensations, including the felt sensation of emotions, much like carefully listening to the unfolding flow of music. Rather than hearing music as background, we can listen to its nuance. We can listen for the distinct sound of each instrument, the force and contour of the notes and musical phrases, the melody, rhythms, bass, and percussion—noticing when one of these becomes foreground or fades, joins others in harmony or discord. Tuning in does more than enhance our listening experience; it transforms it. Similarly, dropping down into the feeling body—each nook and cranny—enhances a felt sense of our immediate experience of being alive.

Discovering Ways In

Discovering *ways in* to the inwardly felt body brings us into an intimacy with life where time opens and one feels "here," situated within oneself, in the present moment. That experience may be comfortable or uncomfortable, but when one can fully enter it, time opens. The theme of the poem in the epigraph *The Way In* elicits questions—perhaps most significantly, the way into what? For me, the poem does not answer that question but rather takes me into an inquiry on that question and others. This inquiry unfolds as I muse on the poem:

The way in—I hear as in to the depth of felt experience. *Sometimes the way in to milk and honey is through the body*, I hear as, *sometimes the way in*, "to nourish life"[2] is through the fundamental substance of milk and the refined substance of honey. Milk is fundamental. It is there from the beginning of our life. Like all other life, ours begins with eating, and we must continue eating to sustain life. This keeps us irrefutably in ongoing interdependence with the earth and all of life. Honey goes through a process of refinement, and we eat it "to nourish life." "To nourish life" is to go beyond feeding the objective body, unsettling the seductive division between body and the spirit—for if *the way in* "to feed one's life" is *a song*, as the poem suggests—this is not reductively terrestrial, and it resists tilting toward the celestial as well. If "my life" is understood as "vital potential," perhaps the poet is offering a guide to nourishing and sustaining this vital potential. She alerts us to the dangerous, to wounding, and to beauty. Life is risky. To love inevitably wounds. Yet she dares us to touch life's beauty because, through this, one can recreate oneself.

The poet also offers us strategies or acts—approaches to responsiveness—which recreate self. She says, "*To enter stone, be water/ To rise through hard earth be plant/ desiring sunlight, believing in water/ To enter fire, be dry...*" By remaining alert, in resonance with the essential qualities of life, such responsiveness, as symbolically rendered by the poet, might constantly replenish our vital potential. We can differentiate from the world by paradoxically resonating with it in unexpected ways.

She says, "*To enter life, be food,*" suggesting that nourishing life in these ways might guide us in nourishing others and the world.

The poem opens me to something unanswerable—something I can't pin down. It could be all of these things, yet it could be something more. When a few words such as—"*The way in*"—open me to so many possibilities, I believe they are a creation of beauty.

Our Brain Dwells in Our Body as Well as in Our Head

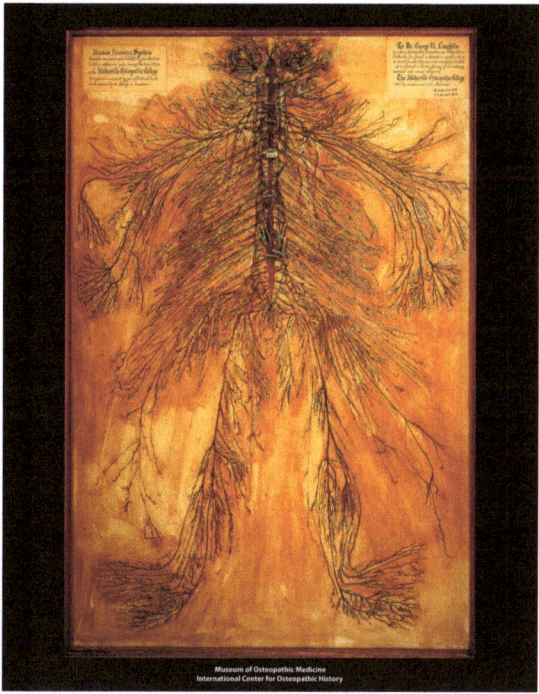

Figure 1.1 An intact nervous system from the base of the brain downward (With permission of the Museum of Osteopathic Medicine)

The brain is both embodied and relational (Seigel, 2022), and not solely an information processor residing in our head. Though we tend to think of the brain as located in our head, our brain also dwells in our body. In fact, we have three "brains," or parallel distributed processing networks, Dan Siegel explains, "one around the gut, one around the heart, and one in the head" (2022, p. 89).

In the embryo, the neural tube is the origin of our nervous system. It becomes the spinal cord, sending out neurons connecting all our organs and forming in complex ways inside the head. The spinal cord is like a moist thick tap root that plunges from the cranium through the torso, finely feathering out, in and around the heart, guts, and organs, shooting through shoulders and hips, then thickly spreading feathery tendrils down arms, hands, fingers, thighs, lower legs, feet, and toes. This intricate network is much like a complex root system that extends throughout the body, comprising the embodied brain.

Sensations are our brain's way of perceiving within our body. This is a paradigmatic shift away from the formulation of meaning-making as an activity occurring solely in the head. As Thomas Fuchs puts it, there is no Cartesian theater resid-ing somewhere in the brain necessary for the body's way of knowing to become conscious—perceptions of the deep body (interoception, see Chapter 2) emerge as consciousness.

When I feel a tingling of air on the soles of my feet, legs, the length of my thighs, the back of my hands, and rounds of my cheeks and ears, my organism is directly informed. In a nanosecond, these stimuli are further transmitted to regions of the brain residing in my head, which then further informs my organism. In turning to receive what my body perceived this morning in my walk, an enlivened hum sang through me. I felt it just as I heard the mountain singing with the rain.

Emotions, too, become known through sensation, first directly in the deep body, followed by the complex intermingling of one's direct experience and the as-sociative meanings elicited in the cortex. Of course, what is distilled from that combining is more than one process alone can render. Our brain is more than an information processor and more than subjective experience.

Scientific understanding of the complexity of how and what our bodies perceive is always expanding and being adjusted. For example, recent studies in neurosci-ence point to our sensory-motor system as the origin of language formation rather than the earlier notion that there is a language center in the brain (Tian et al., 2020; Gallese & Lakoff, in Stern, 2010, p. 49).

Listening to what it is our bodies know is a central theme of this book. Listen-ing to the body as a direct source of knowledge shifts the emphasis of meaning-making away from something primarily derived from language and symbolization. It requires dedicated sensitivity to dis-embed this kind of meaning from the verbal flow more common in talk therapy (Stern, 2010, p. 127). This book will explore the many *ways in* to that kind of knowing, and discover the many dimensions of the "*in*" so encountered.

Though we have this scientific understanding of our brain and mind as embodied and relational, we strongly lean toward privileging psyche to be within our head rather than in our guts, heart, and hands—much less as a relational process. While understandable, given the enormous amount of synthesis processed in that aspect of the brain located in our head, it can be easy to lose contact with the actual basis of experience, with a felt sense of meaning—if we get lost in a predominantly conceptual way of understanding. Our head "brain" evolved to be in service of the other two "brains" (parallel distributed processing networks) of the heart and the gut (Damasio, 2018). Tremendous knowledge emerges from these regions. We cannot remind ourselves too often to drop down into our *bodily-felt experience* and away from abstraction.

What Is Concealed When the Body Is Missing?

David Michael Levin in his multi-volume work, *The Body's Recollection of Being* (1985), points to how Euro-American tradition has kept a body of understanding in concealment. He argues that not only has that tradition suppressed the life and truth of the body, it has also excluded ancient spiritual teachings—traditions of ancient universal wisdom—which speak in the archetypal and mythopoetic language of the body's deep ontological understanding of Being.

Ancient Universal Wisdom Expressed through the Body

Sometimes the Way In Is a Song, Dance, or Posture of Silence

The universal wisdom that is concealed when bodily-based experience goes unacknowledged is far-reaching. Most cultures have some form of spiritual practice that reorients the individual to a more expanded state of consciousness when their inner world narrows. Universally, body-based practices, including chanting, singing, dancing, music, and meditative silence, have served as modes of transformation. This is found in indigenous cultures as well as the organized religions of Abrahamic and Asian traditions. In the more conventional forms of organized religions these aspects of practice have often been sidelined, but this is less so in the mystical aspects of those traditions.

A tangible example of the power of song is shown in the way that enslaved Africans sustained themselves and persevered through some of the worst imaginable treatment through singing as a part of daily life. This kind of singing arises from some fathomless depth of the body, the soul. Neuroscience teaches us that the act of singing itself mitigates highly charged neural arousal activated by threat (Porges, 2019). The words and meaning of songs carry hope, courage, and inspire fortitude, reminding one that they are not suffering and forgotten, alone in the universe, but carried by a much larger force. During an event I attended which was part of a larger project exploring the role of the body in spiritual traditions, Vincent and Rosemarie Harding[3] gave us a deeply moving presentation of such songs, describing in depth their meaning—aspects of which often remained hidden to slave holders—and the way these songs helped carry their people through the hells of slavery in America.

The many kinds of practice, be it song, dance, or silent meditation, facilitate linking[4] the individual to a greater sense of self, to community, earth, and the life force. Each tradition, in its own way, responds to a human need to find reorientation from a constricted self and to offer a path toward wise maturation. Each cultural approach adds nuance that expands and deepens our perceptions of the possibility of the human experience.

Intrinsic to most of these wisdom traditions, whether explicitly articulated or not, is what depth psychotherapy would conceptualize as the development of a self-reflective or witnessing capacity. It is the capacity to self-reflect or witness that makes it possible to accept and work with the transient nature of affective states and beliefs rather than unconscious identification with suffering. When tension and dammed-up energy are caught in our bodily being, what will put us back in the flow of life? No matter what the particularities of the practices, this underlying need—a longing for a state of presence that opens us to the numinous, a longing to belong, and a need for guidance in becoming a wise human being—is ever present in all of them. However, for centuries under the predominance of patriarchal reign, the inner states sought to privilege that which transcends material life, including the body and the earth, in a quest for spirit.

What Is Revealed When the Body Is Acknowledged?

In Western culture, over the last several decades, practices have emerged that are rediscovering the wisdom of body-based knowing. Drawing from centuries of wisdom traditions, this emergent pull toward an embodied knowing arises in various practices and methods. It is informed by traditional approaches that focus on self-knowledge attained through fostering an inner landscape which brings one into a state of receptivity with an essential sense of self or what David Michael Levin refers to as being (1985). This urge to know and live from a more rooted place has for decades (perhaps always) been breaking through the structures of traditional practices and religions. It seemingly wants to be known and takes form in a plethora of ways.

The Emergence of Contemporary Approaches to Bodily-based Wisdom

In the early 1900s new approaches to being with the subjectively experienced body arose, spearheaded largely by women. Elsa Gindler's work, for example, focused on sensing the lived experience of the person moving and exercising rather than the accomplishment of the exercise for its own sake (Weaver, 2015).

Lillemor Johnson worked with touch to literally hear the ebbs and flow of emotion in the cells of bodily tissue, while Gerda Boyeson founded Biodynamic Psychotherapy. Charlotte Selver pioneered the practice of Sensory Awareness. Ilsa Middendorf and Carola Speeds focused on Breath Work. Aadel Bülow-Hansen's refined massage methods co-ordinating breathing, relaxation, and emotional release, and Marion Rosen's work used sensitive touch oriented toward bringing awareness to affective states that dwelled in the body. Bonnie Bainbridge Cohen works with developmental movement and the subtle intelligence of bodily systems. Emilie Conrad Da'oud focused on the effect of micromovements on consciousness. Ida Rolf developed a brilliant approach to structural integration with an eye toward health of the whole person through manual manipulation of the body's fascial system.

These foundational practices gave birth to another generation of practices such as the approach that focuses on the experienced body in movement and stillness as a way to bridge the unconscious and conscious of Mary Whitehouse, which has become known as Authentic Movement, and Gabrielle Roth's Five Rhythms. These, in turn, gave birth to the next generation of approaches, again shaped by women, such as Soul Motion and Body Tales. The lists continue to grow. While there were a few approaches developed by men, such as F. M. Alexander's Alexander Technique, Moshe Feldenkreis's Awareness through Movement, and Stanislaus Grof's Holotrophic

Breathwork, which made important contributions to this movement, it is important to note the predominance of women and significance of their influence.

The 1981 book by L. E. Moss, *A Woman's Way: A Feminist Approach to Body Psychotherapy*, highlights the enormous contribution these women made as they circumvented the patriarchal top-down, logos, left-brain dominant approach to knowledge. As is in keeping with a more right-brain way of knowing—the right brain being the hemisphere oriented to sensation, image, emotion, and nonlinear processing—these women focused on the experiential nature of their work and passed it on orally. Only a relatively small amount of writing was and has been done. The unfortunate result of this is that though these approaches laid an important foundation for a body-based approach to knowing, they remain less known to most (Johnson, 1995).

In the early 20th century, many of these women were central to the fertile dialogue and collaboration that formed the basis of the body-oriented psychoanalysis which arose in Berlin and Western Europe. Much of what has been written about the creative thinking and work that emerged in that time is by the men who were either medical doctors or psychoanalysts, notably Fenichel, Braatøy, and Reich (Bassal & Heller, 2015). What continues to grow forth from the somewhat invisible roots of these women's contributions is the recognition that the subjectively experienced body is central to healing, well-being, and an expanded sense of self.

Inhabiting Our Bodies and, by Means of That, the World

Our bodies carry a fundamental paradox regarding the nature of personhood: Self as separate and self as interrelated. In utero, we are utterly dependent upon our mother. At birth, when the umbilical cord is cut, the distinct boundary of our body largely demarcates our separateness. Simultaneously, we begin to breathe. Breathing, an act essential for life, is accomplished solely by oneself. Eating, also essential, continues but only in relationship with the mother or caretaker. In many ways, nursing or needing to be nourished by another is a hallmark of our mammalian, relational selves. As development progresses, one is soon able to eat by oneself, yet the food comes from other forms of life, from plants and animals. Though breathing is an autonomous action, breathing itself is also fundamentally relational. It is another form of communing with life, life beyond the mother. Plant photosynthesis creates oxygen which we need and inhale. Once metabolized in our bodies it is exhaled in the form of carbon dioxide, which plants require for the photosynthesis process that provides their nourishment. In short, plants help humans breathe by providing us with oxygen, and humans help plants breathe by providing them with carbon dioxide. Rilke expresses the relational mystery of breath in *Sonnets to Orpheus* (Part 2, No. 1):

Breathe, invisible poem!
Always looking after individual being,

Pure exchange of space. Balance,
in which I experience my rhythm.

Sole waves, whose
eventual sea I am;
Most sparing of all possible seas—
Gaining more space.

How many of these spaces were already
inside me? Many breezes
are like my son.
Air, do you know me, still full of my former places?
You once smooth bark,
Curve and leaf of my words.

(Rilke, 1922, unpublished 2024 translation by R. Tyminski)

Our Living Organism as a Spatially Extended Subjectivity

The word psyche is derived from the ancient Greek psyche, "to blow" or "breath of life." Later Plato conceptualized psyche as soul, the immaterial animator of life dwelling in the body. David Michael Levin (1985) poses the question: What are we to make of psyche understood as breath as well as psyche understood as "soul," "spirit," and "self?" Our bodies express a mysterious paradox. Though our bodies seem solid, they themselves are made of atoms held together by certain elusive forces or energy patterns. This kind of energetic dynamics is matched in the field outside the body. "In the ultimate sense, the space outside the body and the space that the body *occupies* are not separate" (Tulku, 1977, p. 54). In certain states of deep relaxation, our awareness expands beyond the literal boundaries of our bodies, and we feel as though internal and external space are one (Tulku, 1977). Here again, one *way in* is through breathing. Thomas Fuchs speaks of our whole living organism as a spatially extended subjectivity. A view of persons not as self-contained monads but rather as inhabiting our body and, by means of that, the world. In so doing, he situates our primary experience in its rightful place again, namely as incarnated beings in the world (2018).

Linking and De-linking Body and Mind

The Body as the Locus of Direct Experience

While the theoretical strivings of depth psychology to understand the inner dynamics of psyche, of the self and self-in-relationship, are invaluable, mind de-linked from body is problematic. As compelling and creative as our thinking capacity is, whether applied to psyche or other realms of inquiry, it can get away from us, leaving us untethered from the texture of life, from the fullness of selfhood housed in our bodies, from others and from our earthen home. We only need look at how our earth is on the brink of being uninhabitable for evidence of this danger. No matter the discipline of inquiry, we have plenty of ideas but need much coaxing to stay with our immediate experience, which is right here, calling for our attention, be it pain or well-being—in us, in the other, or between us and the other, including the more-than-human others of the earth community.

What we call our minds seem to need what we call our bodies in a way that is hard for us to surrender to. Bodies can be messy, uncomfortable, painful, diseased, and feel outside of our conscious control. Yet, they are the source of our direct experiences of love, connection, empathy, reciprocity, awe—the only way we can be present for all that matters to us is through bodily life.

Any Endeavor Can Connect or Alternately De-Link Body and Mind

That we tend to disconnect body and mind is, at least in some part, an aspect of the human condition. Even when one's intent is otherwise, our mind easily races ahead of the immediacy of bodily-felt experience. Any endeavor can connect or alternately de-link body and mind, whether one is conscious of this or not. One may simply inquire within while doing the most common of tasks. For example, when stretching, ask: *Am I stretching the leg*? Or *am I stretching and feeling the sensations of my leg as it interrelates throughout other areas and inner domains*, knowing those sensations are mine, belong to me, versus to *the leg*? Or, while eating, one could inquire: *am I eating*? Or *am I feeding myself*? The body can so easily become the object of our doing mind rather than the place we abide. Charlotte Selver, the pioneering founder of Sensory Awareness, often posed simple questions like: "Is your breath there for your tasting?" or "Are you there for your breath?" Movement and even breath can take us into felt emotion or distract us from felt emotion. Simple lines of inquiry may include: "In movement, are you going with, staying with, feeling, or moving away from it?" or "Is your breath supporting your feeling of sadness?" When the link between the felt sense of emotion and one's attention severs, one's body is no longer the locus of direct experience. A dissociative process may focus one ever more deeply on isolated sensations while disconnecting one from felt emotion. Alternately, a dissociative process may obscure awareness of one's body altogether. Or the body may become an object of the mind. All too frequently, it is a mind that demands a mechanistic perfection of body to transcend emotional vulnerabilities, recapitulating an internalized patriarchal valuing of mental consciousness over embodied life. Even a meditation practice, in which one intentionally focuses on the breath moving in and out the nose, can perpetuate a disconnect from the body and instead reinforce the tendency to make the body and breath *do* as the head prescribes (Ray, 2006). For the dancer or athlete trained to focus on technique, performance, and achievement, the body can become even more of an object of the mind that must conform and perform rather than a place one inhabits and turns toward as the basis of being in the living moment.

Mind–Body Disruption and Development

That our mind races ahead of our body is certainly not new or bound by Western culture.

The Japanese philosopher Yuasa (1987) posit that:

- There is a unity of mind–body intrinsic at birth.
- Disruption of mind–body unity is a typical aspect of human development.
- Cultivation of mind–body unity enhances consciousness and psycho-physical and spiritual well-being.

When things go well enough developmentally, this model offers a helpful perspective.

Adding a Depth Psychological perspective further posits that:

- Disruption of mind–body unity is exacerbated by psychological injuries, insults, and trauma, as well as neurological diversity and those differently-abled, both physically and mentally.
- Psychological injuries and insults can occur anywhere along the developmental perspective, including perinatally.
- Cultural and socioeconomic forces entwine with development, hindering, or supporting it.
- Psychological injury incurred through cultural and socioeconomic forces is enormous and includes transgenerational and current oppression.

Yuasa speaks out of the older Asian traditions of self-cultivation. Self-cultivation is used here as a metaphor borrowed from gardening, referring to the body–mind practices which persons engage in to further inner growth. He elucidates how a few Zen masters in the 18th century strove to make a course correction to the meditative practices, which had strayed away from the recognition that consciousness can only genuinely be enhanced when thoroughly grounded in and through the body. This teaching we find arising again in contemporary meditation teachers such as Reggie Ray (2008) and Willa Blythe Baker (2021) from the Tibetan Buddhist tradition, and Tara Brach (2021) from the Vipassana tradition, who remind us that historically, in Buddhist meditation, the body was the vessel for transformation.

The Body as the Vessel for Transformation

Yuasa (1987) strove for a comparative philosophy that respects the fundamental divergence between Eastern and Western thought while still encouraging meaningful dialogue. In it, they underscore Western intellectual history's focus on the abnormal, diseased, or "universal" (unexamined) human have been concerned with empirical correlations between mental and somatic phenomena, whereas the Asian focus historically centered on those who engage in disciplined practices of cultivating consciousness in order to attain a state of embodiment that *furthers what one is born with*. The recognition that practices that further inner development of body–mind integration can make profound contributions to healing of both acute suffering as well as in elevating the quality of everyday life is typically missing in Western perspectives of psychosomatic medicine.[5]

Self-Cultivation and Self-Care Catalyze the Psychotherapy Process

In Western culture today, there is a growing emphasis on self-care. Generally, this refers to making some time for being nurtured by un-busied time, caring for body and mind through moments of quiet, meditation, contemplative body-based practices, physical exercise, singing, or simply listening to music. In my experience, some ongoing form of self-care not only supports but also catalyzes the psychotherapy process. Yet psychological wounds interfere with one's ability to engage in self-care. Part of the psychotherapeutic process is to soften, dissolve, or learn to relate to the obstacles that keep one from valuing oneself. Comparing Western practices of self-care to Asian practices of self-cultivation overlap can be found, yet "self-care" often drifts toward repairing gaps arising from early negligence or wounds—giving to oneself what is or has been missing or has been inadequate in one's life. Asian approaches to self-cultivation, on the other hand, relate the self to the earth and cosmos and hold a prospective thrust aimed at tending to a maturational process. Yuasa details how statements from the *Bodhicitta Sasta* such as "immediately authenticating the great awakening in the body your parents gave you," emphasize the meaning of attaining bliss in one's actual body in this world rather than just in the quickness of this lifetime (1987, p. 149).

A contemporary interpersonal neurobiological view on a disciplined integration of both, as found in practices such as Vipassana meditation, yields a perspective on the psychophysical basis of spiritual practice. The neurological system engages when we bring *attention* to intention. When one is attuning to the intentional state of another person, such as a parent to a child or therapist to a patient, a state of *interpersonal* attunement is created. When one brings attention to one's own intention, such as in the practice of following one's breath in meditation, a state of *intrapersonal* attunement is created. These states engender the deep sensations of fullness and stability that occur with resonant and harmonious states of mind. These states of interpersonal and intrapersonal attunement promote internal security and coherence in one's sense of self, as is characteristic of secure attachment (Siegel, 2007, pp. 172–173).

A Way In *through Wounding and Beauty*

Jung's approach to the psychotherapeutic process, unlike Freud's, not only looked to address the wounds of the past but also held a prospective orientation, which he termed individuation (1965). In this way, Jung shared a similar orientation toward health as posed by Yuasa, emphasizing the benefit of developing a capacity to self-reflect, differentiate from a state of unconscious merger with the collective, and engage in purposeful modes of becoming a more conscious human being. Holding both poles simultaneously—attending to one's brokenness while also expanding and deepening into one's potential—forges a way toward individuation, *a way in through wounding and beauty*. This is the heart of healing. Here the pain of the past goes through a transformative process, in part through beauty as undefended emotional truth where we enter the present moment and the *next* present moment, which, no matter how laced with sorrow or joy, opens, yet again, to the *next* present moment—into an immediacy of, and an intimacy with life—one's genuine feelings, perceptions, and inquiry. We begin to track the energy flow between us and the other—both other humans and the earth itself—its intrinsic, unsentimental, and sometimes harsh elegance. The opening poem by Linda Hogan speaks of the multiplicity of ways into a deeper kind of knowing. There is no one individual, one culture or psychological approach that holds the only entrance key, just as there is no state that one can attain that captures all of what it means to be a fully conscious human—each culture and approach shapes a facet of the gem of humanness.

Simple, internal shifts of awareness in breathing, or found by entering stillness, silent gesture, conscious movement or sounding, can become gateways to transformative states.[6] When the mind's incessant stream of thoughts quiets, one gains entry to experiencing the living present, where time seems to open, and one feels one is a part of time rather than a bystander to its onward rushing. Body, mind, and emotions align here in a similar way that artists and craft persons find when creativity flows or athletes find when they enter their zone of peak performance. Sometimes numinous experiences of unity ignite, and insight further opens. At other times *mysterium tremendum et fascinosum* takes us to our knees, awed by beauty or terror.

Sometimes the Way In Is Dangerous

The Fast

In Edmonton, Canada, there is a healing center that draws from contemporary methods of psychotherapy and psychiatry alongside traditional approaches to the healing arts of the Native American Cree and other peoples of that extended region. Maggie Hodgson has been instrumental in its establishment and continuance. It serves as a resource for people of that community who struggle with the stuff of daily life, as well as addiction and post-traumatic stress syndrome (PTSD)—an ongoing residue of the devastating effects of colonialism on native peoples. My husband and I have been invited to participate in a five-day fasting ceremony. Maggie and one of the elders here participated in a small group that we had been connected with and that had been convened by the Lifwynn Foundation to explore addiction from a multicultural perspective analysis of the "here and now" of the group. Lifwynn was founded by Trigant Burrow,[7] one of the psychoanalysts who explored the interplay of body–mind, particularly the eye, in the 1930s. There are about twelve individuals who will be fasting. Some are serving time in prison for criminal offenses, some struggle with PTSD, addiction, depression, or anxiety, and some long to be reinspired in their daily lives by the gifts the old traditions offer.

It is early autumn. We will be fasting without food or water for five full days, each in our solo campsite along the wide flood plain of a river in northwest Canada. After an initial sweat ceremony, we are accompanied to our site by the two tribal elders who will oversee the fast. As we walk along the wide flood plain, I am aware of the many young birch saplings that have snapped or been cut. While this isn't so unusual in such a wide flood plain where wind frequently gales upstream, it pulls on my attention. I don't know what to make of the cuttings. I reflect on my privilege and the gratitude I feel for having spent time in many deep wilderness regions that have been protected from incursion and misuse. I reflect on the dark reality of my potentially having greater access to that kind of wildland than the people who were its original inhabitants. Upon arriving at our respective sites, we each make a circular shelter from branches of the abundant low-lying willows that grow along the river, a sturdy tarp, and tie cords. Throughout the fasting ceremony, others of the community will stay in a central house a small distance away, participating in preparations and sweat ceremonies to support those fasting.

I have done several fasting solos in the wilderness before, but never without water and never with indigenous peoples in their traditional way. Also, this is my first time camping in such a northern land. I am not afraid, but I am not, not afraid. What equalizes us as a group is the unknown before us. While this is the truth of any "next" moment, this situation highlights that reality.

It is late afternoon of our second day out. Our only instructions are to stay awake all night and sleep during the day. The afternoon sun is blaring down on my little shelter. There are also a couple of flies that have gotten inside, buzzing about incessantly. The air is dense. It feels like there is a low-pressure system, such as that which typically precedes a storm, laying heavily above the land. Inwardly, I feel unsettled. Hunger and thirst are present, but these have drifted to the background of my attention. I am very aware of feeling sleep-deprived, yet as much as I would like to stay inside and sleep, I am uncomfortable and agitated in a way that is disorienting and hard to deal with. When I lie down inside the shelter it is too hot, and I find it difficult to breathe. Outside, shaded from the intense angle of sun, it is too cold. A wind has come up, and river-bed sand swirls in the gusts. Perhaps it is the flies that have the final say, driving me out of my little abode. I find a place to sit, close my eyes, breathe, and try to settle into a more meditative state. That fails, so I try to quiet my inner and outer agitation by simply becoming a silent observer of the natural world. Five or so minutes pass and the winds gust. I hear a loud crack, and before I quite know what is happening, a tree near me falls directly onto my little shelter, crushing it! I have the inner sensations of being completely emptied from heart to toe: Astonished! Had I not gotten out when I did, I would have been seriously injured, if not killed. The sun is beginning to set, and I know I must rebuild a shelter for myself before dark and possible rain. I gather myself, though still shaking, and begin to clear the debris, salvaging what remains usable. In the shadowy dusk light, I see the elders appear as they round the bend of trail. They have come to make an evening visit. Listening to my account of what has happened, both are quiet, then nod their heads. Their gleaming dark eyes look quietly into mine and let me know verbally and non-verbally, that I had listened well. Had I known something I did not know I knew? Their way of seeing me helps me to see myself more clearly. I settle a bit more into my breath, belly, and legs. With some help, the shelter is rebuilt just before the night envelops the day. Not long after the elders leave, I hear chanting and song emanating from the sweat lodge about a quarter mile away. Each night the community does a sweat lodge ceremony in support of those of us out on the fast. The rhythmic sound of their voices pierce my heart. Their support is the antithesis of what I grew up with and what I experience in my culture. Tears well and fall, softening the long night before me.

There is such complexity in this Fasting Ceremony. A fundamental aspect is the disruption of normal bodily rhythms of eating, drinking, and sleeping. All of these are turned upside down. Our intentions, prayers, songs, and relationships fill the places emptied of food, water, sleep, and contact. As the dark night unfolds, the northern lights dance like beings of light in the night sky. I am humbled; all muscular effort has let down, and I feel gravity's gentle tug holding me to the earth. I feel a great sense of gratitude toward the earth, its beauty and mercy, and toward those present and past who are dear to me. A subtle stream of excitement begins to dance in my heart, filling my limbs with joy.

Synesthesia

Multimodal sensory perception gathers information which registers just below conscious awareness. Each sense modality—seeing, hearing, smelling, touching, being touched, taste, kinesthesia, sense of the presence of others, sense of an inner world—draws cues on an ongoing basis from the inner and outer environment, even though much of that information doesn't reach cognitive awareness in a distinct manner. The perceptual fullness of that gathering is much more than any one mode alone discerns. This multimodal perception is fundamental to intuition. Though language exponentially expands communication it can also foreclose on perception. I think this was so in my experience of the "flies" in my shelter. Naming them "flies," along with my irritation, gave rise to judgment of them as a nuisance, which foreclosed my curiosity about them. To my benefit this did not stop them from buzzing in a rather maddening way. Given that mind, perception, and language are potentially participatory, interrelated process, it is possible that the interaction between the flies and me, the air pressure touching and bearing down on my respiratory process, my earlier attention to the beleaguered saplings, and other non-human elements I was "listening" to, though languaged in a way I did not recognize, saved my life. David Abrams writes:

> Direct, prereflective perception is inherently synaesthetic, participatory, and animistic, disclosing the things and elements that surround us not as inert objects

but as expressive subjects, entities, powers, potencies. And yet most of us seem, today, very far from such experience. Trees rarely, if ever, speak to us; animals no longer approach us as emissaries from alien zones of intelligence; the sun and the moon no longer draw prayers from us but seem to arc blindly across the sky.

(1996, p. 45)

Jung, also spoke of our isolation from nature, underlining this as a source of our psychological disruption: "No voices now speak to man from stones, plants and animals, nor does he speak to them believing they can hear. ...This enormous loss is compensated for by the symbols in our dreams" (Jung, 1964, p. 95). The enormous ecological crisis we find ourselves in makes very clear that compensation of symbolic process, as compelling as it is, cannot compensate the loss of vital earthen life.

Sometimes the *Way In* Is Wounding

Psychological Distress Is Embodied

The upsurge in body-based practices mentioned earlier opened pathways into expanded experiences of well-being but also shed new light on how psychological distress is embodied. Somatic psychology, as a relatively young field of academic study in North America, arose primarily because of the need for psychological training to deal with the prevalence of the complex psychological dynamics that arose from delving into the experienced body.[8] Peter Levine, Pat Ogden, Don Hanlon Johnson, and I all at one time practiced the Rolf Method of Structural Integration. Encountering the psychophysical expressions of trauma that arose from attuned, intimate, deep focused work with the body, sent us looking for ever more comprehensive and integrative ways of working.

Emotions Manifest in the Body as Sensation

Psychological wounds, with their concomitant instinctual protective tendencies, more often than not steer us toward a disavowal of inner pain. Emotions and emotional pain manifests in the body as sensation, though most people are not consciously aware of the sensorial basis of emotion. Disavowal of emotional pain can disconnect us from the felt immediacy of the bodily basis of these wounds. Western culture's emphasis on cognitive understanding merges with the individual's neurological wiring to fight, flight, and freeze in the face of threat, amplifying a disembodied way of life. This disembodied way of life has become the cultural norm.

The Body Is Foreground in American Culture in a Highly Objectified, Subjectively Disembodied Way

The further we are from direct experience of our bodies, the greater that neglected part calls for our attention. This might manifest as tightness, muscular pain,

numbing, over- or under-eating, and addictions of all kinds. The needed yet disavowed calls from our body for attention to emotionally based, bodily experience, is
compensated by externalization of beauty, fitness, health, sex, and pleasure, all of
which are capitalized on by industry's insatiable hunger for profit.

> The less the body is experienced, the more it becomes an appearance; the less
> reality it has, the more it must be undressed or dressed up; the less it is one's
> own known body, the further away it moves from anything to do with one's self.
>
> (Whitehouse, 1958, p. 45)

Thus, the body is foregrounded in our culture but in a highly objectified, subjectively disembodied way. The individual embedded in Western culture tends to not
have an awareness of personal disembodiment. The tendency lives in the region of
what some neuroscientists describe as the non-conscious, meaning it is not unconscious because it has not been conscious and then repressed, but because it is an
unreflected-upon aspect of our reality that hums through our daily existence.

A Brief History of the Body in Depth Psychology

Looking back, we can trace Depth Psychology's early practitioners observing the
body's involvement in psychological distress. Franz Anton Mesmer (1734–1815)
hypothesized blockage of vital fluids that moved through our organism (which he
perceived to be in relationship with planetary bodies) as the basis of psychosomatic
disorders (Marlock, 2015, p. 84–85). Wilhelm Reich (1897–1957) used the term
"Orgone" energy to describe what he saw as the electrical energetic charge that
flowed through people. The perception of energy flow and its blockage in the human organism can be traced back at least as far as the Indian Vedic texts, which in
1000 BC describe the chakras or energy centers in the body. Energy flow through
meridian systems is also central to traditional Chinese medicine and the associated
martial arts such as Qigong and Tai Chi. Prior to Reich, Pierre Janet observed that
distorted breathing patterns and muscular constriction were persistently present
in those suffering with dissociative and other psychological disturbances. In 1929
Janet wrote:

> A new physiological psychology replaces the earlier idea of personality as a
> metaphysical (disembodied) soul. Personality cannot be found in such a notion
> of soul but in the body. By becoming aware of the body, personality is discov-
> ered … We feel our body, we feel our skin, we feel the warmth of the body,
> we feel the inner organs; and this organization of sensations in relation to our
> body gives us our personality. The characteristic features of personality—unity,
> identity, differentiation—are rooted in characteristics of the body … It is not
> possible to progress with the study of personality without first understanding
> what it means to possess a body.
>
> (Janet in Boadella, 1997)

Janet's use of touch to release muscular constriction in the body influenced Freud in his early work:

> Freud had originally worked directly on the client's body, in the form of touch and massage … for Freud the meaning and function of pressure and touch were primarily oriented toward confronting his patients' resistance. This was the entrée for Reich's later work in Character-Analytic Vegetotherapy.
>
> (Marlock, 2015, p. 87)

This integral approach to mind and body was in keeping with the early understanding of Breuer & Freud that the disavowal of painful affects associated with traumatic events formed the basis of emotional disturbance (1895). Freud later repudiated that formulation, adopting instead a theory of neurosis arising from intrapsychic conflict between instinctual drives and the ego. With this turn, the emphasis on the involvement of the body in the repression of unbearable affect shifted, privileging insight over emotional expression. This marked a very significant shift away from the immediacy of *felt subjective* experience to a more abstracted focus on inner conflicts on the part of the analyst, and thus the patient as well (Marlock, 2015, p. 88).

To Rise through Hard Earth, Be Plant, Desiring Sunlight, Believing in Water

After the rise of the National Socialist Party in Vienna in 1933, several prominent psychoanalysts immigrated to Oslo, Norway. Between 1934 and 1939, Oslo became a hub of thinking and exploration about the body–mind relationship in the practice of psychotherapy. A great deal of cross-fertilization unfolded between psychoanalysts, psychologists, physicians, physiotherapists, dance therapists, and vegeotherapists. Their explorations were strongly influenced by the work of Elsa Gindler. At that time Gindler's work fell under the title of Gymnastik, though she herself referred to her approach as "Work with Humans" (1995/1926). Gindler's work focused on the subjectively-felt experience of life in the body, such as breathing, the sensorial experience of posture, muscular constriction, or flow in movement, and how all this was affected by inner emotional life. Gindler lived and worked in Berlin, where some analysts studied with her, prior to moving to Oslo (Weaver, 2015). Claire Fenichel (1981), continued to teach her work after moving, and presented this work to the Psychoanalytic Institute in Oslo. Her husband, psychoanalyst Otto Fenichel, presented on how to integrate certain aspects of Gindler's work into a psychotherapeutic approach. He also authored an article discussing how Freud's "motoric ego" interacts with muscle tone and breathing (1928). Reich settled in Oslo in 1933 and lived there until 1939. His second wife, Elsa Lindenberg, was steeped in dance and also influenced by Gindler's approach (as had been his first wife, Annie). The immediacy of the subjectively experienced body, derived through Gindler's work, and the awareness of posture, breathing, and movement brought forth by those who studied dance, furthered rich dialogue about psychoanalytic technique. Collaboration and debate spurred others, notably psychoanalyst/physician Trygve BraatØy (1954), who conducted research on bio-mechanics and its implication on the mind, into analytic work on the couch. Physiotherapist Aadel Bülow-Hansen's work led to a refined approach that integrated work with breath, movement, posture, touch, and emotional awareness to regulate affective states. Reich, though a complicated and controversial figure, was a passionate force in that movement and remains the most well known. His writings, *Character Analysis* (1933) and *The Mass Psychology of Fascism* (1946) express some of his particular, though perhaps troubled, genius.[9]

Many others who were significant in that creative upswell include Fritz and Laura Perls, Gerda Geddes, and Gerda Boyeson (Bassal & Heller, 2015). The robust community of pioneers articulating the role of the body in Depth Psychology was severely disrupted by the rise of fascism, the Second World War, and Communism. Even at this much later date, we are still gathering many of the lost fragments of genius—a manifestation of the embodied scars of that time. It seems that this work, in its care and attention to the subjectively lived self, stood in opposition to the inhuman objectification that unfolded during the Second World War. The tension of the opposites was held by these and others that prevailed through that time. Now, with the increased understanding arising from infant research, trauma studies, evolutionary biology, and neuroscience, the field is taking up the body in a renewed way.

Bringing the body into Depth Psychotherapy gives further access to that which been concealed by the dominant tradition. The collision of the inner protective mechanisms that attempt to shield us from emotional pain, along with the cultural pattern of disavowing subjectively-felt bodily life, not only disconnects us from painful, unwanted feelings but also keeps us from fully experiencing what is desired: relational repair, warmth, intimacy, love, vitality, ecstatic and expanded states of psychophysical consciousness, depth of pleasure, satisfaction, experiential meaning, and sense of well-being. Experienced meaning arises from full embodiment of emotions and feeling-toned states—savoring positive inner states as well as accepting and working through those that are difficult and undesired (Gendlin, 1981). Consciously working through difficulty can ultimately give way to a sense of well-being, a longed-for sense of wholeness. Something emerges—a something that feels like an opening rather than a constriction—an opening that heretofore was inaccessible. A feeling of constraint lifted can open one into a sense of being with something bigger than the familiar ego identification.

Because the psycho-physical ramifications of trauma can be extremely challenging to integrate, they tend to quickly retreat from daily consciousness. An old phrase popularized by Bessel Van der Kolk, "the body keeps the score," speaks to this in a way that captures something we have known for a long time but which we have had a hard time translating into a rational logic. For years many practitioners have been following the body's logic and found highly effective, if not very idiosyncratic ways of clinically engaging the body's expression of psychological reality (Johnson, 1983). Neuroscience has substantiated many of those carefully tracked lines of response to the most vexing aspects of trauma.

To Enter Fire, Be Dry. To Enter Life, Be Food

While working with the psychophysiological manifestations of trauma does contribute a great deal to healing trauma, I believe the full value arises when this work is added to Depth Psychology's attention to the emergence of mythopoetic meaning and its embodiment. This meaning-making is an intrinsic aspect of being human. It is, as James Hillman (1975) puts it, what transforms life's events into soul-making experiences. However, if a Depth Psychotherapeutic approach pays insufficient attention to the body, the highly charged instinctual responses to traumatic threat that unfold prior to cognition or emotion can remain concealed (Porges, 2019). The psyche's complex story-making function, in tandem with powerful psychological protective mechanisms, attempts to make meaning and to understand these disturbing experiences. In so doing psychophysical responses are frequently overridden, obscuring contact with significant aspects of trauma. What remains in the wake of these incomplete attempts to heal can be a mix of a web of story, which though laced with mythic themes never quite furthers one's moving on and into the difficult arenas of life affected by the trauma. Along with these stories are deep-seated traumatic beliefs and rigid defensive structures which live in, and further haunt the body. Sorting through these complicated threads and strands of trauma will be taken up in case material throughout this book.

Depth Psychology Addresses Which Body and Whose?

Attention to the body can cut to a core sense of experience. Depth Psychology, in its attention to the unconscious, recognizes there are many different aspects of oneself. One of the questions Depth Psychology addresses is: which body and whose? Who am I at any one moment? How is that expressed in my body? Am I able to come into an integrative coherent sense-of-self while navigating the currents that will inevitably send me, once again, into internal disarray? In that process can I find and re-find the potential seeds of creative reconstitution, of self-renewal? Perceiving the psyche's self-organizing and self-regulating capacity, Jung spoke poetically of the psyche's inherent thrust toward growth. Seigel takes up this theme articulating how our minds have an innate movement toward integration and healing. However, trauma interrupts neural integration, moving our minds toward chaos and rigidification.

> An over-emphasis on logical, linguistic, linear, and literal thinking may tilt the balance of our minds away from the important sensorimotor, holistic, autobiographical, stress-reducing, image-based self-regulatory function of our nonverbal neural modes of processing …. Abstract ideas symbolized by words can also make it difficult for us to sense the "lived" details of our human experience. Such experiential knowing is often created best through direct experience.
> (Siegel, 2006, Foreword, pp. xiiv–xiv, in *Trauma and the Body*, Ogden, P., Minton, K., & Pain, C.)

Accessing that central drive toward wholeness and well-being is one of the central goals of individuation. Within this thrust toward wholeness is the psyche's capacity for self-regulation. As we focus on the many different manifestations of self and domains of the mind within the context of an empathic therapeutic dyad, from a neuropsychological perspective, "we enable new states of coherence to develop as neural integration—the physiological linkage of the widely distributed neural patterns in the brain and body-proper—evolve and new forms of healthy, adaptive self-regulation are established" (Siegel 2006, pp. xiv–xv).

As new experiences emerge, new neuro-network pathways are laid down. The more frequently these new neuro-networks are engaged the more they become integrated into an internal working schema. When an individual, having had a new experience, moves yet again into an inevitable state characterized by contraction, brought on by old wounds activated in the normal course of life, the all-too familiar wounded state will now have access to new possibilities. A new path of response exists, the highly charged activation has been mitigated and choice now exists that can further emotional regulation verses automaticity.

This process can be represented by the image of a spiral that depicts the journey through life. In my office hangs a large old African robe. It is predominantly indigo blue. A light-colored spiral is hand-worked into the material. It emerges from a mandala that lies in the center of this beautiful vestment. The mandala contains a four-quadrant square held in a circle. The spiral emerges from the circle. If the robe were worn, the spiral would cover the whole body. Just at the apex of the shoulder the spiral ends in a heart. For me it depicts the long work of life's journey also described by medieval European alchemists, culminating in a heart-centered state of being. That this heart lies on the shoulder—falling at times toward one's front or at times toward the back, or balanced there between, speaks to me of that heart-centered space as one that bridges the past and the present, life and death. To arrive at such a bridge is a worthy fulfillment of a life. To cross that bridge is to relate to oneself and others with heart, where empathy, compassion, and collaboration are possibilities. For me, this is a worthy goal of the individuation process, the term Jung used to depict the goal of analysis: a life oriented toward meaning and self-knowledge.

Over time one learns that as much as one might like to reach one's goal, the end point is a transitory place. We land there only to again circle away from, yet paradoxically that moving away from can be a moving toward, yet again. Beside the robe in my office being very ascetically pleasing in its evocation of a profundity cleanly and simply depicted, I appreciate that the spiral covers the whole body, implicating our whole-life and whole-bodied-self in this endeavor.

Body–Mind?

I have not found an adequate term in the English language that communicates the unity of psyche and body. The word *person* has its etymological roots in Greek referring to mask. However, there was a time when the word *body* signified "the material being of man as the sign and tangible part of his individuality, taken for the whole": the "person." *Body* has commonly been used interchangeably with *person* to refer to a human being regardless the sex, and has been combined with *any*, *every*, *no*, and *some*. *Body* is derived from the Anglo-Saxon *bodig* and the Old High German *botah*. It is also derived from the German *bottich*, which means cask, vat, or brewing tub, suggesting that the body is the alchemical vessel where the subtle processes of transformation unfold. Here sensation, sensory motor processes, movement, stillness, gesture, beauty, pain, and symptoms are the way in and through. As these bodily activities unfold, affect comes into play as well as image. And consciousness of one's experience and the meaning of that arises from sorting and sifting through the mix. For some, it is the body and its ongoing reality, rife with pleasure and pain, symptom and well-being, that tethers them to the reality of the psyche, the humility of life on earth. Our organisms are a microcosm of the universe, infinitely complex, expanding and contracting, all the while our feet have only this ground. It is those moments of entering the extraordinary ordinariness of life, when we experience what is described as interpersonal neurobiology—our minds as embodied relational processes right here, with others and the earth. These are moments in which we are infused with a sense of beauty and belonging that makes the hard work of life, of transforming suffering, worth living.

In the 17th century the new science initiated by Newton, Galileo, and Descartes needed a clean distinction between the realms of body, mind, and spirit to enable the new science to develop free of the religious authority that had constrained the earlier unfolding of human inquiry. They argued that the body as an object being measurable was the realm of science, while the interior realms of the "subjective body" were left to theology and religious authority. The rigid side effects of that liberatory divide became a defining perspective of the Enlightenment period. The unforeseen side effect of objectification of the human body had far-reaching ramifications. One of the most horrific was justification to indulge in the slave trade. Concomitant with this was the boon and misery of the industrial revolution. Now, one's laboring body no longer belonged to its person, robbing life of one's own sense of time, depriving one of needed respect, connection, and the sense of belonging that gives meaning (Johnson, 1983). The concept "body–mind" is inadequate for undoing the Cartesian split that plagues us. As much now as then, this inner severance is perpetuated because of disparity of wealth, institutionalized racism and the transgenerational pain that haunts our socioeconomic structures.

We are left with these glaring questions: Can we learn to give bodies back to their persons? Can we learn to re-inhabit our bodies by reclaiming the rights to our subjective bodily experience? Can we actualize the recognition of the rights of others to do so as well? I believe we must before the conjuncted word mind–body can begin to communicate real meaning.

Despite the many vectors of theoretical consideration, for me, psyche—as soul—when spoken with its etymological Greek roots, gets close to expressing the unity of mind–body as it links psyche to life which unfolds in the body. However, this, too is complicated. Plato posited that the spirit leaves the body at death. The Abrahamic religions strongly privilege spirit over matter as do the Gnostics, though the emphasis differs in each sect. Indigenous cultures commonly perceive all forms of life, including what Westerners believe to be inanimate, to be imbued with soul or spirit. Many African and other indigenous cultures believe the spirit leaves the body at death. However, this must not be confused with the Western dualism that separates physical form from spiritual. This idea comes to life in the poem *Breaths*, by Birago Diop, an African American whose poems are rooted in oral African traditions. Ysaye Maria Barnwell adapted the poem to song, which she sang with the ensemble Sweet Honey in the Rock. The song and original poem call on us to listen more often to things than to beings, to listen for the breath of our ancestors in the voice of fire and water. It gives a tangible reality to the perception that our ancestors are not under the earth but inhabiting the elements of the earth—the groaning rocks and trees, the flickering fire, and the sound of the water. In this way, they establish the continuity of life after death, including the body's life.

The attitudes expressed in this poem-song are in kinship with those of deep ecology, recognizing that at death, the body is reborn. From the perspective of deep ecology, the (un-embalmed) body too, whether cremated or buried, decomposes into elements that contribute to the nourishment of all life, be it that which teems in the soil, eventually becoming intrinsic to the food we eat and air that we breathe, or other facets of the greater eco-system of the whole earth community.

All these pages are my attempt to lay down some of the weight of Western religious and philosophical history that hovers about us. Because of this, in the common use of the word "psyche," the split between mind and body persists, and the body goes missing in most psychological discussions. In this book, I will use various conjunctions and sometimes psyche or *soul* to refer to body–mind unity.

The Turn toward Moment-to-Moment in-the-Body Sensing and Feeling

Over the last few decades numerous psychoanalysts have made valuable contributions to this struggle of how to help us think about and be with the mind–body.[10] The thrust of this book is a turn toward the *body as experienced*. Slowly, perhaps for some reluctantly, there is a warming up to be with the body as experienced in the moment-to-moment unfolding of the analytic encounter—be it in the body of the analyst or the patient.

In that turn toward experience, multiple therapeutic modalities have emerged that attempt to bring experiential distant concepts experientially near. For example, Jung conceptualized the archetypal Self, a concept distinct from ego in that it is the archetypal (typical) self-organizing principle of the psyche rooted in the collective unconscious. Yet, for some, this can seem abstract—experientially distant. Experiential modalities have honed in on the psychic reality alluded to in the term the "Self," such as Hakomi's "Essence" (Weiss, Johanson & Monda, 2015), Internal Family Systems' term the "Larger Self" (Schwartz, 2021) and the "Core State" construct of Accelerated Experiential Dynamic Psychotherapy (AEDP) to name a few. Each of these are experientially based psychotherapeutic modalities. Each gets at some part of what Jung theorized.

Jung himself spoke of analysis being nothing if not an experience (1943/1966). However, many people stray away from Jung because it seems too conceptual. A deep experience is what happens in the best of an analysis. But not all. Gendlin (1996) illuminated how psychic transformation occurs in shifting attention away from cognition and toward the felt sense. The felt sense can be described as moment-to-moment in-the-body *sensing and feeling*. Such a shift in focus accesses the wisdom of the body and its natural healing processes rooted in adaptive strivings and self-regulating functions.

The relational turn in psychoanalysis creates the foundational basis of this moment-to-moment experience in the affectively alive analytic couple. Turning further inward toward a deeper stratum of experience, toward inwardly experienced body-based sensations, of both the analyst and analysand furthers that endeavor. Learning to stay with bodily-based experience can feel analogous to relating to Proteus' shape-shifting. Sensations are mercurial, shifting in and out of attentional foreground. Sometimes from heart to gut in a nanosecond, sometimes from a vague cloud of numbness to a pulsing, difficult-to-contain level of activation in the chest and face. Or a tingling in the hands and arms leading to hyperventilation, which triggers survival panic. These not-so-comfortable, capricious states can easily keep the therapist from entering or pursuing what may quickly seem uncontrollable and thus unhelpful. Unfortunately, straying away from these somatic quickenings can foreclose on aliveness and lead to therapeutic impasse.

Both Freud and Jung, each in very different ways, strove to articulate how the inner world was dynamically related to the body. As I have outlined above, much has unfolded since their time that helps bring that bridge between the body and the inner world of the psyche into focus. Numerous psychological thinkers and a few Jungians continue to build that bridge through their writings. This book is my contribution to that bridge. I imagine it as a bridge emerging from the mists in an ancient Chinese painting. If you look closely, you see places where construction is not yet complete, and other sites intricately carved. It may never be fully completed, yet it holds an eternal home in our desire to know. Many years ago, an artist and dear friend of mine, Rosalyn Driscoll, whose work is dedicated to expressing the subjective experience of being a body, curated a show at the museum in Brattleboro, VT. The title of the exhibit was *The Body Imagined through Time and Culture*. This question of how the body is experienced and imagined has and will reverberate in just that way—through time and culture.[11]

Notes

1 The concept of "presence" has a particular prominence in Asian martial arts. The one who embodies such a state commands a dynamic power of being—that is, one who does not easily lose themselves but rather is grounded, awake, alert, attuned to, and highly responsive to her surroundings; empowered. Such a practitioner will be highly adept at her art. "Real Presence" in the Christian tradition refers to the real presence of Jesus Christ in the Eucharist.

2 The work of Francois Jullien (2007), by juxtaposing Western philosophy's tendency to categorize mind distinct from the body as well as the sacred as transcendent rather than

immanent, to very early Chinese philosophy, has, along with the native American poet Linda Hogan, been of great help to me.

3 Vincent Harding was an African American pastor, historian and scholar who authored multiple books, including *Martin Luther King: The Inconvenient Hero* and *Is America Possible*. He also drafted Martin Luther King Jr.'s speech, "A Time to Break Silence." His rich and varied work included serving as chairperson of the *Veterans of Hope Project: A Center for the Study of Religion and Democratic Renewal*, at the Iliff School of Theology. Rosemarie Harding was a community activist, social worker and Feldenkrais practitioner. The immanent knowledge of the body was foundational to her work. The Hardings co-founded Mennonite House, an interracial voluntary service center and movement gathering place in Atlanta, GA.

4 The origin of religion is derived from *religare*: re (again) and *ligare* (bind, link or connect).

5 See Dossey's (1985) perspective on the foundations of healing based more on quality of life than riddance of disease.

6 See Van Loben Sels, *The Shamanic Dimensions of Psychotherapy*, for a discussion of gesture, movement, singing, drumming, and silence—ancient attributes employed for experiences of transformation.

7 Based on his work with eye movement associated with emotional disruption, Burrow has been considered the grandfather of Eye Movement Desensitization and Reprocessing (EMDR). He also pioneered work with groups emphasizing analysis of the "here and now" unfolding.

8 See Don Hanlon Johnson's (1983) discussion of this in *The Body and Psychotherarpy*.

9 See Buntig (2015), "The Work of Wilhelm Reich, Part 1: Reich, Freud, and Character," and Young (2015) "The Work of Wilhelm Reich, Part 2: Reich in Norway and America," both in Marlock et al. (Eds.). *The Handbook of Body Psychotherapy and somatic psychology*,

10 See Harrang, Tillotson, & Winters (2022), *Body as Psychoanalytic Object: Clinical Applications from Winnicott to Bion and Beyond*; Aron & Anderson (2000), *Relational Perspectives on the Body*; Anderson (2007), *Bodies in Treatment*; Orbach (2009), *Bodies*; Lombardi (2017), *Body–Mind Dissociation in Psychoanalysis: Development after Bion*; Ramos (2004), *The Psyche of the Body: A Jungian Approach to Psychosomatics*; Sidoli (2000), *When the Body Speaks: The Archetypes in the Body*; Chodorow (1991), *Dance Therapy and Depth Psychology: The Moving Imagination*.

11 See "Body, The." *New Dictionary of the History of Ideas*. Encyclopedia.com: www.encyclopedia.com/history/dictionaries-thesauruses-pictures-and-press-releases/body (retrieved December 11, 2023).

References

Abrams, D. (1996). *The spell of the sensuous: Perception and language in a more-than-human world*. New York: Pantheon Books, p. 45.

Baker, W. B. (2021). *The wakeful body: Somatic mindfulness as a path to freedom*. Boulder, CO: Shambala Publications.

Bassal, N., & Heller, M. C. (2015). The Norwegian tradition of body psychotherapy: A golden age in Oslo. In G. Marlock, H. Weiss, C. Young, & M. Soth (Eds.), *The handbook of body psychotherapy and somatic psychology* (pp. 62–70). Berkeley, CA: North Atlantic Books.

Bateson, G. (1972). *Steps to an ecology of mind: Collected essays in anthropology, psychiatry, evolution and epistemology*, cited in Fuchs, T. (2018). *Ecology of the Brain*. Oxford: Oxford University Press.

Boadella, D. (1997). Awakening sensibility, recovering motility: Psycho-physical synthesis at the foundations of body psychotherapy: The 100 year legacy of Pierre Janet (1859–1947). *International Journal of Psychotherapy, 2*(1), 45–56.

Braatøy, T. (1954). *The fundamentals of psychoanalytic technique: A fresh appraisal of the methods of psychotherapy.* New York: John Wiley & Sons.

Brach, T. (2021). *Trusting the gold: Uncovering your natural goodness.* Louisville, CO: Sounds True.

Breuer, J., & Freud, S. (2000/1895). *Studies in hysteria.* New York: Basic Books.

Damasio, A. R. (2018). *The strange order of things: Life, feeling, and the making of cultures.* New York: Pantheon.

Dossey, L. (1985). The future of medicine. In D. Kunz (Ed.), *Spiritual aspects of the healing arts.* Wheaton, IL: The Theosophical Publishing House.

Fenichel, C. N. (1981). From the early years of the Gindler work, in *The Charlotte Selver Foundation Bulletin: Elsa Gindler, 1885–1961, 10*(2), 4–9.

Fenichel, O. (1928). Organ libidinization accompanying the defense against drives. In H. Fenichel (Ed.), *O. Fenichel: The collected papers of Otto Fenichel, 1st Series* (pp. 128–146). New York: W. W. Norton.

Fuchs, T. (2018). *Ecology of the Brain.* Oxford: Oxford University Press.

Gendlin, E. (1981/1978) *Focusing.* New York: Bantam Publishing.

———— (1996). *Focusing-oriented psychotherapy: A manual of the experiential method.* New York: Guilford Press.

Gindler, E. (1995/1926). Gymnastik for people whose lives are full of activity. In D. H. Johnson (Ed.), *Bone, breath, and gesture: Practices of embodiment* (pp. 5–14). Berkeley, CA: North Atlantic Books.

Harrang, C., Tillotson, D., & Winters, N.C. (Eds.). (2022). *Body as psychoanalytic object: Clinical applications from Winnicott to Bion and beyond.* London & New York: Routledge.

Heidegger, M. (2008). *Being and time.* New York: HarperCollins.

Hillman, J. (1975). *Re-visioning psychology.* New York: Harper & Row.

Hogan, L. (2008). *Rounding the human corners.* Minneapolis, MN: Coffee House Press.

Johnson, D. H. (1983). *Body.* Boston, MA: Beacon Press.

———— (1995). *Bone, breath and gesture: Practices of embodiment.* Berkeley, CA: North Atlantic Books.

Jullien, F. (2007). *Vital nourishment: Departing from happiness.* Brooklyn, NY: Zone Books, Urzone.

Jung, C. G. (1943/1966). On the psychology of the unconscious, in *Two Essays on Analytic Psychology.* CW 7.

————1964. Approaching the unconscious. In *Man and his symbols* (p. 95). New York: Doubleday.

———— 1965. *Memories, dreams, reflections.* A. Jaffé (Ed.) & R. Winston (Trans.). New York: Random House.

Levin, D. M. (1985). *The body's recollection of being: Phenomenological psychology and the deconstruction of nihilism.* London: Routledge.

Marlock, G. (2015). Body psychotherapy as a major tradition of modern depth psychology. In G. Marlock, H. Weiss, C. Young, & M. Soth (Eds.), *The handbook of body psychotherapy and somatic psychology.* Berkeley, CA: North Atlantic Books.

Marlock, G., & Weiss, H. (2015). Preface: The field of body psychotherapy. In G. Marlock, H. Weiss, C. Young, & M. Soth (Eds.), *The handbook of body psychotherapy and somatic psychology.* Berkeley, CA: North Atlantic Books.

Marlock, H. Weiss, C. Young, & M. Soth (Eds.) (2015). *The handbook of body psychotherapy and somatic psychology.* Berkeley, CA: North Atlantic Books.

Moss, L. E. (1981). *A woman's way: A feminist approach to body psychotherapy.* Yellow Springs, OH: The Union for Experimenting Colleges and Universities.

Porges, S. (2019). Rethinking trauma: Polyvagal theory can revolutionize your work with trauma survivors. An interview with Ruth Bucznski at the National Institute for the Clinical Application of Behavioral Medicine. https://s3.amazonaws.com/nicabm-stealthseminar/Rethinking-trauma-new/Stephen/NICABM-StephenPorges_Part5-Transcript.pdf

Ray, R. (2006). Touching enlightenment. *Tricycle: The Buddhist Review.* Spring 2006.

——— (2008). *Touching enlightenment: Finding realization in the body.* Louisville, CO: Sounds True.

Reich, W. (1972/1933) *Character analysis.* New York: Farrar, Straus & Giroux.

——— (1970/1946) *The mass psychology of fascism.* New York: Farrar, Straus & Giroux.

Rilke, R. M. (1922). *Die Gedichte.* Vierte Auflage. Insel Verlag, Frankfurt am Main (Germany).

Schwartz, R. (2021). The Larger Self. IFS Institute. https://ifs-institute.com/resources/articles/larger-self

Siegel, D. J. (2006). Series Editor's Foreword. In *Trauma and the Body: A sensorimotor approach to psychotherapy.* New York & London: W. W. Norton & Co.

——— 2007). *The mindful brain: Reflection and attunement in the cultivation of well-being.* New York: W.W. Norton & Co.

——— (2022). *IntraConnected: MWe (Me + We) as the Integration of Self, Identity, and Belonging.* New York: W. W. Norton & Co.

Stern, D. B. (2010). *Partners in thought: Working with unformulated experience, dissociation, and enactment.* New York, London: Routledge.

Tian, L., Chen, H., Zhao, W., Wu, J., Zhang, Q., De, A., Leppänen, P., Cong, F., & Parviainen, T. (2020). The role of motor system in action-related language comprehension in L1 and L2: An fMRI study. *Brain and language 201.* https://doi.org/10.1016/j.bandl.2019.104714

Tulku, T. (1977). *Gesture of balance: A guide to self-healing and meditation.* Berkely, CA: Dharma Publishing.

Weaver, J. O. (2015). The influence of Elsa Gindler. In G. Marlock, H. Weiss, C. Young, & M. Soth (Eds.), *The handbook of body psychotherapy and somatic psychology.* Berkeley, CA: North Atlantic Books.

Weiss, H., Johanson, G., & Monda, L. (2015). *Hakomi mindfulness-centered somatic psychotherapy: A comprehensive guide to theory and practice.* New York: W. W. Norton & Co.

Whitehouse, M. (1995/1958). The Tao of the body. In P. Pallaro (Ed.), *Authentic movement: Essays by Mary Starks Whitehouse, Janet Adler, and Joan Chodorow.* London: Jessica Kingsley Publisher.

Yuasa, Y. (1987). *The body: Toward an eastern mind–body theory.* Kasulis, T. P. (Ed. & Trans.), Albany, NY: State University of New York Press.

Chapter 2

Sensing the Self, Sensing the World

The Primal Feeling of Being Alive: Interoception

> If we fancy some strong emotion, and then try to abstract from our consciousness all the feelings of its bodily symptoms, we find we have nothing left behind, no "mind-stuff" out of which the emotion can be constituted, and that a cold and neutral state of intellectual perception is all that remains ... A purely disembodied human emotion is a nonentity.
>
> (William James, *Principles of Psychology*, Vol. 2)

My own direct experience, and a form of a "sort-of-knowing," a kind of implicit knowledge that has been percolating to consciousness over many years, has compelled me to continue to explore the premise of the primacy of the body from multiple points of view. Neuroscience offers one "way in" to think about and illuminate what we feel, or in some cases, do not feel, in our bodies. While cognitive neuroscience has largely neglected the cyclical interaction between body and mind, affective neuroscientists, particularly Damasio (1995, 1999), and Panskepp (1998a, 1998b), perceive a primary subcortical origin of consciousness (Fuchs, 2018). Their research posits that the primary existential felt sense of being alive arises from the deep body—whether this is felt as a state of well-being or malaise. It is known through the experience of our heart beating, blood pulsing, breath moving, guts working, hormones shifting, heat rising, cold spreading, hunger and thirst demanding, and through sexual arousals announcing themselves (Fuchs, 2018). This is the interoceptive system. It is comprised of our deep viscera and nervous system which, in constant interaction, constitute our organism's self-regulatory process of homeostasis. This moment-to-moment, back-and-forth interaction registers within as our deepest source of feeling. Whether felt as an existential state of well-being or discomfort, these feelings belong solely to oneself and arise from the body. This direct, embodied experience provides a feeling of ownership. Through this, I know my experience is my own, and my feelings are mine. Interoception affords us a sense of who we are. Damasio posits this as the very origin of consciousness.[1] All feelings have their foundations here. Feelings are a representation of what is going on in the body at any moment.

DOI: 10.4324/9781003305804-3

Feelings let the mind know, automatically, without any questions being asked, that mind and body are together, each belonging to the other. The classic void that has separated physical bodies from mental phenomena is naturally bridged thanks to feelings … Self-reference is not an optional feature of feeling but a defining, indispensable one.

(Damasio, 2021, p. 78)

These homostatic, subcortical experiences are instinctual, impulse-driven. This primal sense-of-self, which Damasio refers to as the protoself (1999), is furthered by basic felt instincts and corresponding motivational affects that are crucial for vital and emotional survival: seeking, rage, fear, panic, lust, care, and play. The seeking system generates the arousal which awakens our interest in the surrounding world, fueling our attention. At first, this seeking is undifferentiated and objectless, and only differentiates with experience. Consider an infant searching for nourishment and finding the breast, or later the seeking of sexual partners, or the instinctual seeking of a change in environment. The primal impulse to fight or flee also arises from such an elementary motivational system. We share with all mammals these primary instinctual and affective experiences that guide our living. Again, these basic affects are felt rather than intentionally perceived. In other words:

The self is not a result of cognitive sophistication or reflection: rather, it arises with the affective and motivational instincts that serve the organism's vital needs. The role of the cortex consists in establishing the intentional direction of basic affective consciousness to external objects. This happens both in the dimension of cognition and emotion. (To note, we are not yet dealing here with a reflective or "ego" experience, which only arises on the third level of the autobiographical self).

(Fuchs, 2018, pp. 115–116)

An affective neuroscientific perspective understands that psyche is embodied and could not be otherwise. The level of primary subjectivity so far discussed is originally pre-reflective. It informs us at a basic level as to whether we feel well or not so well. Many people develop reflective awareness of some of these underlying bodily-based primal processes. However, others have little such bodily awareness. So, while embodiment has this scientific basis, which becomes elaborated as development proceeds, the notion, as well as the experience of embodiment, is often pondered as if it were a hypothesis, puzzle, or *koan*.[2]

Interoceptive Awareness

Although interoception is often described as simply the sensations that arise from the inner body or as the sensorial elements derived from the organism's homeostatic balancing (Bernston, Gianaros & Tsakiris, 2019), a more detailed description includes the organs, hormonal and neural systems, and their associated processes.

From a psychotherapeutic point of view, distinguishing interoception and *intero-ceptive awareness* is essential as current research points to *interoceptive aware-ness* as affecting a change in consciousness (Sedeño et al., 2014). Interoceptive awareness is what gives rise to a felt sense of embodment. Interoceptive aware-ness refers to an experiential felt sense of one's heart beating, or breath moving, activity in the viscera or surges of hormones such as adrenalin. Very few have continual awareness of these functions or awareness of the entire spectrum of in-teroceptive activity. But the ability to notice and feel one or more of these functions defines interoceptive awareness. Interoceptive awareness can be fostered by inten-tional, mindful awareness of these physiologic states that often lie at the borders of consciousness (Joshi et al., 2021). Doing so brings a felt sense of unity of body and mind. I think it is safe to say that when most psychotherapists talk of embodiment, they are talking about a general awareness of one's body, especially the ability to feel feelings in one's body. A more granular focus reveals that "awareness of and exposure to these often private, physiologic symptoms is an important part of many evidence-based therapies for anxiety disorders" (MacDonald, 2007, p. 51). This significance is further borne out in research that shows clear links between com-promised interoceptive function and psychiatric disorders, including depression (Avery et al., 2014), anxiety (Paulus & Stein, 2010), addiction (May et al., 2014), and depersonalization derealization disorder (Sedeño et al, 2014).

Case Study of Eva

I present the following case study to show how and why focusing on interoceptive awareness became crucial in regulating hyperarousal and developing a reflective capacity to the rapidly shifting self-states that previously remained dissociated for this patient, Eva. While Eva had some degree of interoceptive awareness while meditating, the lack of safety she felt in the world, and with me particularly, ac-tivated a dissociative process. In these times, interoceptive awareness was com-pletely unavailable to her on her own; she needed a co-regulating other to re-find this level of self-awareness. However, others, including myself, are precisely what activated the dissociative process. Thus, her breath became the "way in."

Interoceptive Awareness and Its Disruption in Trauma

While Eva and I had a good analytical relationship, with positive regard and shared fondness, my presence nevertheless stirred an enormous amount of fear rooted in her early history. Our task became to engage her interoceptive layer of experience to bring about co-regulation and enough sense of interpersonal safety that productive therapeutic exploration could further unfold. Over time, our continued attention to this layer of experience, in turn, helped cultivate *interoceptive awareness*, laying the groundwork for affect recognition and tolerance. In contrast, attempts to focus her attention more directly on the emotions engendered between us, whether through attunement, empathic inquiry, or interpretation, only heightened the activation of the pre-reflective states of fight, flight, and dissociation. This kind of chaotic confusion is characteristic of disorganized attachment and the accompanied dissociation of, and between, her rapidly shifting fragments of an early ego self (Payne, Levine & Crane-Godreau, 2015). When sufficient interpersonal safety allows access to what Stephen Porges refers to as the social engagement system, generative psychotherapeutic exploration unfolds (Porges, 2019).

The Story of Eva

There is a lot in Eva's compact stature: wit, pain, shame, sharp perception, childlike joy, excitement, and desire to share. Years of attending extended meditation retreats give her access to states that hold an immediate sense of presence and a knowing of what most do not know about focused attention. Right alongside this are profoundly traumatized states that are far removed from that knowing. There is something she seeks. It guides her like a compass needle that points north and though, at times, she forgets it is in her pocket, the compass continues to function. There is a current of courage within that follows the compass without question, though it, too, usually operates far in the background of her awareness. Typically, her immediate awareness directly contradicts any conscious awareness of that courageous part. She communicates all this, sometimes at a dizzying speed and jumble that lets me know she knows, while denying she knows. The combination entices me. I wish for her to know what she knows, and to discover that, despite the shock and trauma that shattered her capacity to maintain an ongoing coherent sense of self, she is still standing. She is moving toward true north.

Eva is a psychotherapist. Although not always able to acknowledge her abilities, her colleagues respect her keen perception and unflappable presence with clients, especially those struggling with behaviors others find too difficult to deal with. She works in a clinic serving a diverse array of individuals and couples located in the heart of a vibrant San Francisco neighborhood.

Eva came to me well-informed about Jungian Analysis, including working with symbolic processes unfolding through dreams and Active Imagination. The part of her that orients by following her inner compass believed she would be able to grow by working with the relational dynamics engendered through transference. She had engaged in many different healing modalities throughout her life—some partially satisfying, others not so—including psychotherapy and an earlier analysis. Following these, she continued to work with the upwelling of her psychic content through an art therapy group. She and her husband of 27 years were in their late fifties when Eva and I began our work together. Their oldest daughter had gone off to college. Their younger daughter would soon be moving out. Her husband's work required that he travel extensively. With more space opening up in Eva's life she felt ready to do more inner work.

She came wanting to work with a form of Active Imagination, known as Authentic Movement (Pallaro, 1999), that she had not previously explored.[3] In this practice, the body, as experienced in movement and stillness, including the internal stirrings of interoception, is the medium of exploration. She felt that working with inner bodily experience might help work through some of what she referred to, as her social anxiety, and difficult feelings about herself and her body. She yearned to be able to understand and embody the meaning arising from her dreams and art-work. A dream she had in the early phase of our work often entered our conversation. In the dream, a war veteran roams homeless. She first appears walking down the hill at the center where Eva attends meditation retreats. The woman looks Eva directly in the eye, saying "*I was in the war*." Eva and I understood that the dream represents the part of her that needs to find a place inside for the traumatic feelings she carries from the past. The dream expressed how this part of her, which arises into her awareness during her meditation practice, needs containment, a home for the traumatized parts of herself to settle.

We soon learned that it was not yet possible to work with the practice of Active Imagination through movement. The dissociative processes and relentless inner attacks that Eva struggled with rendered that mode of exploration fraught with the potential of re-traumatization. We found that she would become identified with an intense inner pressure to perform that stemmed from internalized, highly unrealistic family expectations for exceptional achievement. She would also experience states of overwhelming psychoneurological activation that made it hard to be with felt sensations. She found it intolerable to be with vulnerable feelings.

She also found it hard to focus inward yet it was often equally frightening to open her eyes and see me. We explored several variations of working with Authentic Movement to accommodate these struggles, but overall, it felt too fraught. The activation, rooted in the trauma she had experienced, needed more safety, attention, and containment. Looking back, she can say, in simple terms, that at the time, she could not tolerate (that is, accept and be with) the unfolding of unpleasant sensations—the basis of emotions too terrible to bear.

On one of the few occasions that we did explore working with Authentic Movement, she encountered a memory too frightening to accept, which she could not talk about until much later. This further highlighted that though she did not consciously recall early trauma, or was dismissive of what she had experienced as having been traumatic, its presence was announced not just by the memory that had arisen but in our ongoing interactions. She knew that the fear she felt in my presence had to do with what it was like for her as a child when with her mother. Still, this understanding did little to quell the difficulty of emotionally accepting how intensely hyperactivated she would become in my presence. As much as she wanted to explore less verbal modes of therapy she was utterly compelled to talk. Davies likens "the attempt to help patients reintegrate early trauma via verbal interpretation, while in a state of physiological hyperarousal, as trying to teach calculus to someone in the middle of a panic attack" (2023, p. 257).

Just knowing that our meetings held the potential to elicit emotions was perceived as dangerous to the traumatized little girl within. For that vulnerable little one, those feelings were to be avoided at all costs. For that little girl, therapy and the therapist (me), were dangerous. This was in direct contrast to the adult part of her that wanted to do analysis, felt safe enough with me, and knew why and what our therapeutic work entailed (Davies & Frawley, 1994).

We decided to set the formal practice of Authentic Movement aside, continuing instead to work with the *principles* of that practice. We would do this within the safety of seated, moment-to-moment dyadic engagement. We would be employing body-based, trauma-informed approaches so that we could slowly titrate the relational activation and emotions she felt. In this way, we would safeguard against re-traumatization by intending not to overwhelm her with more than could be metabolized in the moment. We agreed to rely heavily on the principles from Somatic Experiencing (Levine, 2010), integrating that work into a more relationally based Jungian analytic context (Soth, 2019). It took quite a bit of experience together and negotiation between us to get to this point. Jody Davies captures our dilemma, stating:

> When memories of abuse begin to return during psychotherapy, they do so as physiological bodily states, but also as unintegrated sense memories; smells, tastes, random visual and auditory images. The return of these fragments is almost always accompanied by overwhelming anxiety, a level of terror attached to the original abuse and not to the current psychotherapeutic situation. Such "dissociated affect" calls upon the creative resources of the therapist to help the patient contain these affect storms, at least to a degree that facilitates a slow reprocessing and integration of what is being experienced in the here and now.
>
> (2022, p. 256)

Through a somatically based approach, we were sometimes able to move with and through the sensations and affects that were arising, and she frequently felt nourished by our relational interactions. However, states of high arousal, often activated by a hair trigger, tripped autonomous defensive mechanisms that sought to quell the fear via persistent self-recrimination and persecutory attacks on me, the therapist, or on the therapy. The emotional logic of the defense went something like this: the underlying fear could be avoided if she could control her own or my behavior. Sadly, though, this only induced more anxiety. The vicious cycle of self-protection so common to trauma survivors, is described by Kalsched as the archetypal self-care system (1996, 2013). Archetypal refers to a psychic instinct. In other words, many of us would have a similar instinctive response given a similar context. When this pattern began to be recognized in war veterans, it was likened to hysteria. Trauma expert Peter Levine (2010) refers to it as the trauma vortex.

As Eva and I worked to navigate the choppy waters between us, a vague sketch of her largely dissociated childhood emerged. It took time to metabolize, but she was beginning to realize that even though she had little or no narrative memory, her body remembered, and "What is remembered in the body, is well remembered" (Scarry, 1985, p. 110). She began to understand the need to linger with what was unfolding between us. The following account offers a snapshot of the tumultuous unfolding between us:

> As soon as Eva enters my office, her keen hyper-charged vigilance kicks into action. She picks up even the tiniest signs of difference on my face or in my behavior, which signal to her the potential of danger—a simple greeting versus a smile of welcome, a clearing of my throat, the faintest watering of my eyes. These spark fear and questions as to whether I am sick or an alarming concern that someone has died and that I must have been crying before she entered. Any remark from me other than one that she senses to be authentic elicits an adamant belief that I am not telling her the truth but rather a story that elaborates her suspicion. Though her story does not accurately depict my internal state, she nevertheless, at times, has some uncanny intuition of a detail of my private life. Because her insistence on the validity of her assertions about my inner state can feel intrusive, it compounds our already complicated dynamics. I learned that what worked best was to acknowledge interest in her perceptions, without affirming or denying them, while letting her know that I was interested in her experience through the prosody of my sighs and other nonverbal acts of recognition. However, the feelings of intrusion I experienced could engender anger and impatience, and I, too, could begin to feel hyperactivated.
>
> All this unfolds before Eva has even sat down. Upon entering, she assesses me as she helps herself to some tea. In this process, her anxiety heightens even more. She is compelled to have tea because of the concrete sense of comfort she derives from my providing it, yet simultaneously is seized by terror. Fear that any wrong move on her part will result in an "accident"—a dribble on the carpet or a potential mark on the table where she sets her cup—induces terror. Any attempt to explore this leads to tangential comments that become nearly impossible to contain. Though we eventually came to know the context quite well—it was rooted in the history of being terrorized by a mother who could become profoundly unhinged by an accident such as milk spilled at the dining room table—it still stirred a terrible chaotic fear.
>
> From the time Eva was quite young to well into her teenage years if such an event occurred, her mother would lunge at her and pull her hair. Sometimes Eva could dart away. However, her mother would then chase her, ultimately trapping Eva in her bedroom, where she would proceed to pull Eva's hair—out—and leave her there alone as if nothing had happened. Later, her mother would inevitably ask Eva, in a cheery, sing-song manner, if she wanted one of her favorite things to eat. Eva learned that the best thing to do was to go along with the cheery pretense to avoid things worsening.

Working somatically was the most effective way to contain the flood of emotions that would otherwise be concealed in words. However, what further helped was the occurrence of two synchronous events (Cambray, 2012). On two occasions, Eva's paper cup *did* leak onto the little table she had set it on. She became very upset with me. The weary, fragmented little girl within would quickly shift to a parental, managing role. This part of her would now come on duty to oversee my incompetence, as evidenced by my providing such shoddy cups. All this indicated that she would have to intensify her watch on me and manage my missteps.

On the one hand, these events heightened the beleaguered little girl's fear. Yet these occurrences simultaneously helped the adult in her to *emotionally* take in that her struggle to avoid an accident was much greater than the part of her that desperately tried but inevitably failed to control her behavior. While intellectually, she had understood the need for us to attend to all of this, another part of her just wanted to get on with telling me about the difficulties in her daily life and "not talk about all this transference/countertransference stuff." These synchronistic events confirmed the significance of what was unfolding and highlighted a felt sense of meaning in working with it.

Peter Levine, the founder of Somatic Experiencing, conducted a research project that underlined how avoidance of interoceptive cues only further hinders one's capacity to evaluate the environment; yet focusing on the negative interoceptive signals increases fear reactions (Payne et al., 2015). Eva and I learned over time that once she sits down, the best way for us to work with the activation is through a process in which we purposefully breathe together, during which I verbally support her to focus specifically on her exhalation. To maintain the focus and contain her anxiety, it helped to delineate the specific number of breaths we would take together—usually four. If she is left to direct the amount of breathing we do, her attention will be disrupted by an intrusive associative thought that she is compelled to talk about. If we do much more breathing, it kindles anxiety; if it is too short, it is insufficient to affect a co-regulatory process. As we breathe, I offer verbal guidance for her to carefully track and name the felt sense of the path of the exhalation as well as the accompanying felt sensations of the release of tension.

Tracking and naming the felt sense of the sensations and, if occurring, the relief or increase of tension manifesting in her deep body is key in regulating her distress. Becoming aware of her bodily sensations creates a basis to contain the chaotic flood of emotional activation she tries to manage with words. Because the words cognitively override what is actually going on at the interoceptive level, it worsens the agitation. At the onset of the analysis, when we attempted to explore any of this, she would quip that she did not feel, nor had she been feeling anything underlining the dissociative processes at work.

One of our fundamental tasks has been, and is, to help her develop interoceptive awareness—awareness of the felt sense of her breath, her heart beating, activation in the layers of her skin, especially her limbs, and her inner sense of warmth or coldness. Finding moments of a felt sense of connection through resonant breathing allows her to land in her bodily self and be with me in the room. Bringing sustained awareness to her exhalation facilitates the regulation of overactivation.

Eva's many years of meditating provide a foundation to draw from so that with my help as a co-regulating other, there are times she can attune to her breath and rather quickly enter a state she describes as calm. Sometimes it is a calm that arises from a shift in self-state. She shifts away from the part of her that had been highjacked by fear only moments ago. If this happens, I hold it in my awareness as a pendulation (Levine, 2010) between the two states. However, from a more conventional psychodynamic perspective, the "shift" in self-state could be ascribed to dissociation. Eva and I found that it was too early to verbally explore this process, because engaging in verbal exchange, no matter how directive, would throw her "into it" again. We'd then have to re-establish a base of regulation, rarely a straightforward path.

At other times the state of calm she enters through our breathing together affects a soothing of the previous grip of fear. Regardless of which of these two possibilities unfolds, I understand either of them as a needed regulatory event.

When a regulated base is established, and I inquire further, she has learned to sense and locate where she experiences "calm" in her body—usually in the heart and lung regions of her chest. From here, she can prolong and deepen her felt experience when accompanied by open-ended, *facilitated* guidance. I might ask if she notices a feeling of warmth or coolness (temperature) and how small or large this feels inside. Exploration such as this encourages a spatial sense of unfolding sensation (bringing a sense of continuity, of going on being, to her core sense of self). As her interoceptive awareness comes into focus, in this part of herself that she has heretofore dissociated from, she discovers that she *can* be with herself. From here, she slowly began to formulate her inner experience (Stern, 2019).

Adjunctive Help: Making Art

We arrived at a point in the analysis in which we were meeting three hours a week. However, because of how bumpy this all could be, we discussed what might help us along our way. Amidst the various possibilities, such as some practice that would help her be in her body more consistently, what persistently arose was her desire to express herself creatively. Eva felt drawn to visual art, even though she doubted her capacity for it. She decided to join a small group art class that had roots in depth psychotherapy. Though the same inner dynamics she and I encountered plagued her, some deep current prevailed. The process involved just the right balance of artistic instruction while emphasizing the value of exploration over product. She felt good about the facilitator, and though she struggled with feeling hyperaroused, she grew to feel safe enough in the group. An appreciation for her aesthetic sensibility slowly took root. The work she created there and some of her earlier pieces became essential to her analysis. Some of those images will be incorporated here and again in Chapter 7 where, with the focus on trauma, I will present more of our work together.

Figure 2.1 is a collage painting that Eva did in the art class.

This image symbolically depicts the near-impossible inner tension that she has had to bear, and which plays out between us: the bloody baby nursing at the breast of Medusa (Bright, 2010). It depicts her need to be nourished, yet the mother figure, the source of nourishment, hurts her and is utterly terrifying. Furthermore,

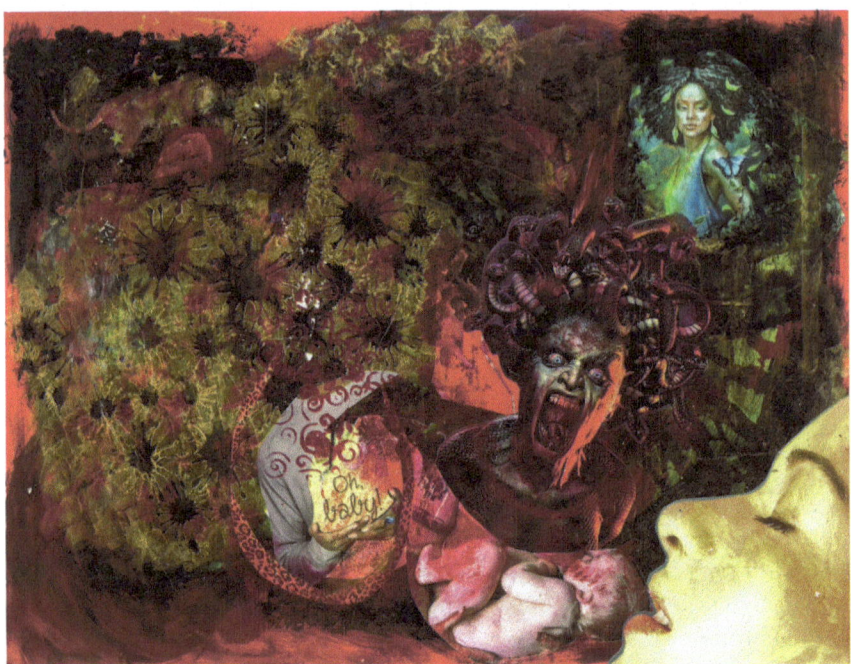

Figure 2.1 Bloodied infant nursing at Medusa's breast (Original artwork by Eva, with permission)

it captures the inner fragmentation depicting a young woman seemingly asleep or unconscious of the situation, and the one (on the bottom left) whose headless body remembers and validates, exclaiming, "*Oh, baby!*"

This vignette illuminates how co-regulation unfolds primarily at the interoceptive layer of experience. Interoceptive awareness, particularly when accessed in relationship, can aid in re-establishing cohesion of the core sense-of-self (Stern, 1985) or the implicit self (Schore, 2011) that is vulnerable to fragmentation by inadequate early caretaking, trauma, and dissociative processes.

Though it is because of our relationship that this co-regulation could unfold, it was also true that my responses at times did frighten her. At times, I would express my frustration and anger at being cut off and disregarded by being talked over. Sometimes my responses were reflective, and, at times, I found it hard to contain the powerful emotions and reflect as much as I might have wished. Sometimes I felt righteous in my reactions; sometimes, I felt a sense of shame at the harsh edge of my unreflected expression. I understood some of my feelings to be solely my own, necessitating my own sustained inner work. At times, some of the feelings I understood as evoked through somatic resonance with a dissociated part of herself, or as a process of projective identification in which I carried the angry and shameful feelings that she could not bear. At other times, I understood those feelings as a complementary countertransference (Racker, 1957). We worked to repair these upsets between us.

In the repair process, it was vital for her to know that it was not my intent to hurt her. If I did hurt her, I would acknowledge, take responsibility for, and reflect on my behavior. Perhaps most important in our process of repairs was that she heard that I had feelings and less-than-perfect parts of myself. While I accepted this and knew this required my ongoing attention, I did not believe it was OK to hurt her. Moreover, when I did, I intended to be accountable and do my best to let her know that the conscious adult in me did not mean to hurt her (Davies, 2023). I wanted to underline that what happened between us was not about her being a shameful bad person. It was something that unfolded between us and required us both to work through.

Working with the somatic aspects of her experience was about more than just helping her physically calm down so we could do analytic work. Interoceptive awareness is significant in building a foundation for affect tolerance. Eva was developing more capacity to feel difficult sensations and thus tolerate emotions that she previously had to dissociate. She was developing an implicit self that was less rigid and more able to flow from one state to another (Schore, 2009).

As we continued along, Eva and I understood her frequent reflection on the homeless wandering veteran was helping her more fully integrate that the little girl within that had *experientially felt as though she had been "in the war"* and had directly experienced trauma. We worked together to help her understand that this was the source of the dissociative chaos she experienced when with me rather than her deep insidious fear that she was "bad."

There seems to be no way for a child to survive physical abuse by a parent other than by splitting into separate self-states (Davies & Frawley, 1994; Davies, 2022). The kind of war zone Eva had endured was torturous. Generally, Eva knew and felt she was cherished and provided for, but she also knew that could change in a split second to terror and torture, which for a child includes being left alone with physical pain and emotional terror—and the direct and indirect denial of it ever having happened. Her dream of the war veteran spoke to the need to heal which she had begun to find in her meditation practice—a need to reconnect and find integration within rather than fragmentation. An innate right to be here rather than to be severed from her body, her feelings, her inner home, and the longed-for sense of presence that occurs as one brings awareness to one's inmost self—the interoceptive elements of dwelling in our bodily being.

The Interoceptive Loop

Pulling the neuroscientific thread forward, interoception is simply the basis of self-experience. It is from this deep-bodied basis of interoception that we meet the world. Within a flash, as our inner chemistry meets the bioelectric currents of the nervous system, feelings, affects, and emotions resound within. Images and associations emerge. Interoception intertwines with exteroception in what Fuchs

(2020) calls the interoceptive loop. Exteroception is our sensorial experience of the world and the others in our world; we see, hear, taste, smell, and touch the textures of engagement. At any moment, emotions arise—be they fear, disgust, or joy—and our hearts may expand, guts cringe, skin crawl, and breathing stall or quicken. These visceral responses beget a new visceral state and a new body–brain interaction, resulting in a feeling that is now partially "emotional" rather than purely homeostatic, begetting yet a new affective state. When sustained over time, such affective states give rise to what we call moods: upbeat or down, dulled or excited with which we begin our day.

For me, being with the body in depth psychotherapy is to attend to this multilayered, moment-to-moment unfolding. Being with this immediacy of the "how" of experience heightens a sense of life lived, a felt sense of feelings. It can also be key in working with psychophysical protective mechanisms, especially the hyper- and hypo-active states engendered in trauma, as shown in further work with Eva.

Attention to Interoceptive Loop While Working with Eva

At times, the process with Eva is much more tumultuous: Her arms flood with intense tingling, triggering the fragmented little girl within who proclaims, as she flaps her hands and swings her lower legs back and forth, that she hates feelings. Naming the little girl's presence, I might remind her that while this is so for the frightened little girl, the adult in her knows the value of being with and working through feelings. Sometimes, this is enough to help her shift from a state of merger with the frightened little girl to an adult state with reflective capacity (Davies & Frawley, 1994). From there, we can work together to titrate the traumatic activation. In this context, titration means to be with her experience of sensations, affects, memories, and images bit by bit, staying within a window of tolerance (Levine, 2010). Because of the strong pull to dissociate, it is important to focus primarily on sensation until there is adequate inner cohesion to do otherwise. Previously, Eva and I have discussed the intention of working this way; it is that of regulation of arousal rather than catharsis and the importance of titrating the intense tingling and feelings rather than overwhelming her again (as happened as a child) with more emotion than she can metabolize—which would only be retraumatizing. Working with these states requires the added exploration of her sensorial experience throughout her musculoskeletal system and skin to titrate the intensity of arousal. Sometimes, these surges of sensation are expressive of a release of tension that had been held inwardly in a state of freeze. If so, I reassuringly name the tingling in her arms as such, assuring her that it is enough to feel a little bit of it. I am aware that, as the tension is transformed, she is able to sense/feel her bodily self rather than be cut off from feeling.

Alternately, when she enters that very young part of herself, characterized by a higher pitched voice, a slight inward turn of her legs and a rapid swinging of her forelegs, I might direct her attention to her legs and feet, simply asking her to attend to the movements that have organically arisen there and inquiring if she can slow them down so she can become conscious of what her body is trying to express. As the swinging movements of her legs slow down, I ask her to notice the sensation in the soles of her feet when they make contact with the ground.

In so doing, I ask if she can just let the action be slow enough to feel it and sense its purpose—perhaps it is an impulse to walk or run. "Run," she quips. *While she remains in her chair*, I encourage her to allow that impulse to run to happen by stepping (in place) and bringing her awareness to the sensations of her foot touching the floor with each "step," again, while she is still in her chair (Levine, 2010). From here, we can explore where, in her memory or imagination, the running might want to take her. She follows this cue in a process I conceive of as active imagination, which incorporates bodily felt sense (Chodorow, 1999) with some guiding principles of Somatic Experiencing. The felt and imagined running breaks through the traumatic terror and thwarted instinctual impulses to run when trapped (Tronick et al., 1978; Levine, 2010).

Alternately, if we cannot help her down-regulate, a term used here to mean dampen or calm the hyperarousal, the session will be flooded with dissociated talk, which is so fast that it rarely allows my voice to enter. This communication style has three conflicting functions: First is the desire to connect; second is a desperate need to give me enough information to help her; third, and unconsciously, it functions to keep me away so I do not hurt her. Toward this end, she will talk, one tangent leading to the next, with no space for me to enter. If I attempt to dialogue in any way, she will talk over me. When she does, with my help, slow down and become conscious of this process, she describes her behavior by quoting Marion Woodman as "Cut off at the neck!" (Woodman, 1987, p. 4). The words are accompanied by a gesture in which her hand is the knife at her neck; the action is swift and not to be questioned. Indeed, this dissociative process disconnects her head and thinking from the rest of her body and, with it, the capacity to feel.

Her positive affection toward Marion Woodman allows us to slow down and reflect on what is happening. Rather than addressing her verbally, her gesture cues me to wonder aloud if she might be able to bring her attention to the inside of her neck and the feel of her breath as it enters her nose and passes through her neck into her chest. Emphasizing awareness of the felt sense in her neck of a slow exhalation again aids in regulating the intense over-activation, which has occurred alongside a freeze response. The felt sense bridges her thoughts and feelings to her experiencing body (Levine, 2010).

As something like the above unfolds, a memory frequently arises, or she recalls a dream that links her bodily dynamics to personal knowledge of her inner world, furthering that sense of ownership that she otherwise reports feeling disconnected from. Alternatively, she may begin a session by laying out her artwork, which depicts the characters and affective states of her inner world. The images can further help her link her experience of the inner parts of herself to the sensorial awareness she is now in touch with. This is crucial as it validates the importance of her work, countering and quieting the inner voice that otherwise intrudes, denies, or dismisses

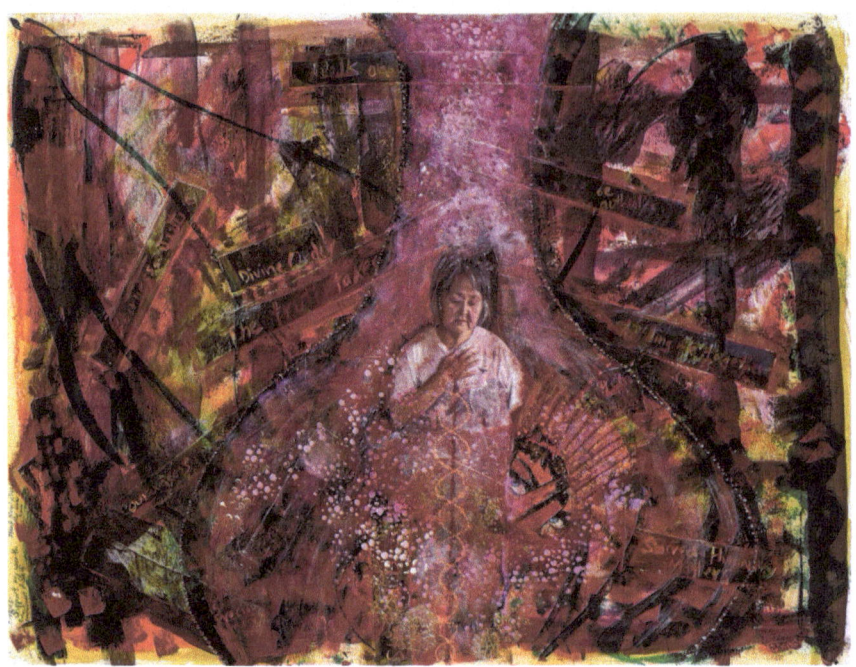

Figure 2.2 The Alembic contains feminine compassion for the terrified, wounded one (Original artwork by Eva, with permission)

the whole endeavor causing her to dissociate again (Davies & Frawley, 1994; Kalsched, 2013). This struggle to stay in her body and work with these very challenging energies and emotions that arise when in my presence is at the heart of her analytic work. Her artwork helps her to voice with images that which was not available to her in words—there was little or no conceptual memory. Her body remembered. As we made a home for those bodily-based memories, her psyche responded, and the images emerged as she engaged in the art process. She did not come with the image in mind unless one had arisen in a dream. Once formulated through the art, the works helped her remember rather than dissociate, further supporting a sense of inner continuity of self (Daniel Stern, 1985) and helping to bring more coherence to what has previously been unformulated (Donnel Stern, 2019).

An Alchemical Vessel Forms through Developing Interoceptive Awareness

Figure 2.2 depicts an Inuit woman whose hand is on her heart as she gazes compassionately down at a figure huddled under her hearth. The figure, which first arose in a dream, is that of a methamphetamine (meth) addict seeking cover near a hearth. In the art-making process, he (recognized by her as an inner aspect of herself) found the place he had been seeking in the Inuit woman's abode. In this piece of Eva's artwork, a mix of collage and layered painting, the scene described is held within an alchemical alembic. For Eva, the meth addict represents this dynamic that has had something like an addictive hold over her to run from this awful arousal and the accompanying feelings, be it with me or in other social interactions. And, because she is aware of the "running," and that it is antithetical to her explicit desire, the behavior induces interpersonal shame.

Eva frequently places this image above the image of the medusa and infant as she works to metabolize the terror induced in my presence. The Inuit woman represents a compassionate woman, whom she initially associated with me, her therapist, whom she felt had consciously known her own suffering. Thus, she could offer compassionate witness to the one in her who is merged with the one who "runs in fear." This would help her to remember and feel, even if fleetingly, that there was the possibility of empathy and compassion for this part of herself rather than feeling lost in shame. Transformation is at work within the alchemical vessel depicted in her collage painting: she holds the opposites of shame and compassion in a generative tension.

Moving back and forth between these images with bodily felt awareness is known in Somatic Experiencing as pendulation. Additionally, from a Jungian perspective, she is bringing pneuma or spirit into matter. The Oxford Dictionary defines *pneuma* as the Greek term for "that which is breathed or blown, the vital spirit or soul of a person." Breathing her spirit into her body relinks what had been severed. Over time, the Inuit woman's gesture became her own. The act of bringing her own hand to her heart and feeling, from the inside out, what it was like to be touched helped her to feel her physicality—and thus feel compassion toward herself truly unfold in her body rather than as an idealized thought or something that had to be supplied by me. With self-touch, one touches and is touched; here, she consciously internalized the therapeutic relationship in a bodily felt way.

Interoceptive Awareness and the Importance of Slowing Down Associative Process

When working with sensorial elements associated with highly activated residues of traumatic experience, slowing down associations, especially interpretations or meaning-making responses, is essential. It is crucial to avoid foreclosing on the unfolding psychophysical process by prematurely attaching a story to the sensation, as this frequently perpetuates cognitive override of body-based experience (Levine, 2010). This vignette details how this unfolded with Eva. When she brought her artwork to a session, we would toggle back and forth, weaving sensorial-emotionally based processing with the images and meanings that arose. While for the most part, the images helped her from dissociating, at other times, they were the vehicle by which she could get away from difficult sensations and emotions. Together we would track what was happening, tacking and readjusting as needed.

Some researchers have found a correlation between interoceptive awareness and a tendency to catastrophize (Sedeño et al., 2014). This might result from shifting away from uncomfortable and unwanted sensorial experiences into meaning-making before the organism has sufficient time for the psychophysical regulatory processes to unfold. For example, when Eva's arms would flood with sensation, the frightened fragmented little girl within did not "like" feelings and intense sensations. The little girl within labeled them as yucky and bad. She typically wanted away from them as quickly as possible. This is why a co-regulating other was essential for Eva, and will often be necessary for most others when processing difficult interoceptive sensations.

It is equally important not to de-link meaning from psychophysical injury as the sensations are psychosomatically processed. Doing so can become a part of a dissociative process. Over-emphasis on sensation and movement can be used to dissociate from emotion. Bringing meaning to bear must be well paced and depends on the psychophysical dynamic at hand. Because Western culture leans so heavily toward conceptual understanding, we frequently need to allow the body-based sensations to be felt before meaning. In this way, the meaning can arise from the direct experience—bottom-up processing rather than from a conceptual or urgent fear-based drive that unfolds top down (Schore, 2009).

A body-informed, depth-psychological approach attends to the unfolding psychophysical processes, including the here-and-now relationship with the analyst. Eva's primary trauma was revivified in our relationship, putting those dynamics front and center. The careful cultivation of interoceptive and exteroceptive awareness facilitated affect tolerance and recognition of affects arising between us. Staying tethered to moment-to-moment experience in a bodily felt way helped her develop self-continuity and self-coherence from states of fragmentation. The mythopoetic expressions were essential in eliciting and deepening a felt sense of personal meaning and bringing cohesion to her autobiographical narrative.

Without the somatic work, she would quickly slide into dissociative conceptual associations when working with dreams and imaginative processes. Kalsched puts it this way: "In some cases of early traumatic injury, there is relational work to be done with embodied emotion, connecting psyche and soma, and opening the imagination, before conventional analytic work can be initiated" (2020).

Exteroception: Meeting the World

The feeling of being alive vivifies as one meets the world. The infant emerges, breathes, and is held. This meeting engages in sensing what lies outside the body. As mentioned before, the term exteroception is used to describe this domain of sensorial perception. While I will describe exteroception as a distinct realm of the somatic senses, its basis is always the interoceptive deep body: The infant breathes, her heart is beating—interoception—and she simultaneously feels the warmth and contact of being held by her caregiver—exteroception. Thomas Fuchs, who approaches psychiatry with a phenomenological and neuro-affective perspective, speaks of "being toward the world" in this way:

> In enactive terms, this corresponds to the structural coupling of organism and environment, produced by *functional cycles of sensorimotor interaction*. Here, the lived body is pre-reflectively experienced as the point of convergence of action and perception. Interoception is the basis of exteroception; the self-affection of the deep body provides the sense of mineness, which pervades all interactions with the world. In this way, basic bodily self-awareness becomes a world-directed, extended consciousness.
>
> (Fuchs, 2020, p. 4, original emphasis)

Through our sensorial experience, we come to know the world. To be touched and to touch the other, to be touched by and to touch the air; the textures of life, whether sharp or velvety, rough or smooth; the sounds, whether harsh or thrilling, jolting, or soothing. All are registered via our sensory perception and we respond through movement—no matter how subtly—toward or away from the source. We smell the one who touches us and are comforted or recoil. We see eyes that welcome and we smile in response, or see eyes whose cruel gaze makes our skin crawl and our chest tighten. We feel the other's contact with our skin. "Sensations occur not only on the surface of the skin but also within the skin, felt as pressure, temperature, and vibration" (Driscoll, 2020, p. 21). Colors and shapes, rhythms, and repose vivify the world we continually discover. We dance with, or curl inward in grief toward, the world. Our emotional experience is coupled with some trace of movement; the word emotion is rooted in the Latin *emovere*, meaning to "move out." Such movements may be highly expressive or a subtle occurrence of muscular activation imperceptible to another or unnoticed even in oneself. Whatever the case, the effect of our sensory experience echoes and blooms throughout every dimension of our psyche. Through our movements and multimodal sensory perceptions, we come to know ourselves.

> Whether on an unconscious, subliminal level or in the full light of attention, our perception of these sensations continuously operates to provide us with a sense of who we are and how we are at any given moment as well as over time. A large part of our identity derives from our movement habits and patterns. They stabilize our sense of self. To explore new movements is to possibly disrupt and to potentially expand our sense of self.
>
> (Driscoll, 2020, p. 50–51)

Children immerse themselves in the world with their bodies. They learn by feeling, smelling, tasting, touching, moving, hearing, and mimicking. Through the nuances of facial expression and bodily resonance, they feel their way into the shared space of relationship and the rhythms of culture. This multimodal sensorial realm of bodily engagement is the very foundation of knowing. It is the way we link to the natural world (Holifield, 2022). It is our basis of relationship with the ordinary, extraordinary earth on which we dwell. Conscious relationship with the earth requires conscious valuing of sensorial experience. To dismiss the significance of the body is, in effect, to dismiss our valuing of the earth.

It is these everyday experiences that thinkers like Merleau-Ponty, Thomas Fuchs, Sabine Koch, Don Hanlon Johnson, Rosalyn Driscol, and David Abram have brought attention to in a world that largely neglects this domain.[4]

The Cultural Shaping of Sensory Perception

All too frequently, Western culture narrows how we conceive of our sensory perception of the world to the five senses of taste, touch, sight, smell, and sound. However, there is a whole realm of sensory perception that shapes our inner experience of the world. The kinesthetic sense refers to the sense of the motion of our outer body known through muscles, joints, and skin. The proprioceptive sense informs us of where we are in space—singular parts and their overall integration as we move. Seigel (2007) includes the inherent way we sense our interconnectedness, that is, how we feel the presence of another in our vicinity even when we neither see nor hear them. In addition, he includes our sense of having an inner world as a primary aspect of sensorial perception. Others also include our sense of the experience of gravity and our sense of up and down.

> The human sensorium ... never exists in a natural state. Humans are social beings, and just as human nature is a product of culture, so is the human sensorium. ... Tastes and sounds and touches are imbued with meanings and carefully hierarchized and regulated so as to express and enforce the social and cosmic order ... Perception is not just a matter of biology, psychology, or personal history but of cultural formation.
>
> (Howes, 1991, pp. 3–4)

For example, the Anlo-Ewe people of Ghana in West Africa derive how they know what they know through their concept of *seselelame*—a concept that embraces emotion and sense perception. *Seselelame* translates into feeling in the body, the flesh or skin, or perceive-perceive-at-flesh-inside. Kathryn Geurts, who conducted extensive ethnographic research with the Anlo-Ewe, found that their sensory order was not limited to the five senses, a concept they perceived as a curious folk tale. Rather than five senses, they orient to *seselelame*, a more overall feeling in the body encompassing internal senses such as proprioception and balance, voice, and other perceptual, emotional, and intuitive dimensions of experience. *Seselelame* is a culturally elaborated manner of how the Anlo-Ewe people attend to their own bodies while simultaneously attuning to the bodies around them. *Seselelame* sometimes refers to a tingling on the skin that might signal impending illness, sexual arousal, heartache, passion, inspiration to dance or speak, or to describe something like intuition. The most tragic loss of sensation for the Anlo-Ewe people would be that of hearing, as loss of this mode of sensual perception would cut one off from others as well as cause disruption to one's sense of balance. For the Anlo-Ewe, interaffectivity is a primary source of knowing and consciousness. This contrasts with Damasio's emphasis on one's individual experience of feeling as substantiation of subjectivity and, thus, the bedrock of consciousness (Geurts, 2005).

Variations in sensorial emphasis are far-reaching, expressing cultures' shape, color, and complexity. For instance, Western culture has, at least since the Enlightenment, long elevated visual perception in a way that seamlessly serves as a basis of mental conceptualization (Driscoll, 2020), while those whose cultures that have remained rooted in earth-based traditions value multimodal sensory perception and kinesthetic perception over cognitive conceptualization. In addition to an embodied emphasis on sensorial modes of perception that differ, a person of a non-dominant culture may also feel a lack of resonance with others in the more dominant culture manifesting as an overall sense of unease that registers as diffuse tension throughout one's body. Discrimination and social injustices heighten that unease and, over generations, give rise to deeply embedded states of persistent hypervigilance (Menakem, 2017).

Case Vignette: Jackson

Jackson is an African American man with whom I worked as he struggled to find his place in this world. He was 32 when we began working together. Jackson taught in a local elementary school. Both faculty and students were of mixed race, culture, and socioeconomic class, yet the surrounding county was predominantly white middle- and upper-middle-class. Jackson's experience was that of not belonging and not feeling "a part of" the school or the greater community. This manifested within as anxiety and social unease. A kind of aggressive competition seeped into his relations with others. He tried to keep this feeling under wraps as it was quite alien to his self-identity.

Jackson had a passion for physically focused activities. However, it also seemed he tried to manage uncomfortable feelings with an intense focus on physical training. His grace and capacities to both do and teach complex movement were extremely satisfying to him yet at another level left him feeling rather alone. While he found a sense of pride in his physical prowess, he was unable to give voice to or appreciate the other parts of his considerable sensitivity. He practiced and taught a form of weight training, postural alignment, and efficiency of movement oriented toward achieving refined strength and the visible results of body shaping.

In part, Jackson sensed that his practice of physical training helped him to come to know himself. Through our work together, he was better able to link his inner subjective experience with his bodily sense of self. The ground had been prepared through his physical training to access felt sensation. Integrating this with his emotional experience occurred in our work together. It seemed to me that, at least in part, when his focus tended to narrow on his body's capacity to perform, it situated him as an object to himself and others, amplifying the barrier that kept him from accessing his own interiority. He in no way flaunted the visual beauty of his body; feeling comfortable with being seen in that way was difficult. However, he got positive attention for his body's beauty, which stirred inner confusion. He longed for respect, acceptance, and love from others, yet without fully knowing it, what he needed was respect and acceptance of his whole self. This could never be fulfilled by being seen in an objectified way, regardless of whether that recognition came from self or others.

Early in our work together, he complained of pain in his right shoulder. The pain became the portal to his interiority. I encouraged him to notice the felt sense of the pain without trying to change it. By staying with and discovering the dimensionality of internally felt sensation—for instance, how the muscular tension felt more like a metal guy wire, fraying because it was strained to its limit, rather than a rope tightening in toward him—he could feel the physical expression of the way he braced himself from a sense of threat that he perpetually guarded against. He began to feel the burden and exhaustion of that constant bracing, and came to understand it as a state of vigilance that he felt had been with him for as long as he could remember.

In time, I inquired, and he revealed how he felt a similar bracing with me, a white woman. As we together found our way to understand and normalize his experience and its basis in the racial prejudice against people with black skin that permeates our world, there was an easing of the restriction in his breathing.

As our work unfolded, he began to speak of pain deep in his solar plexus. We explored that pain and how it radiated from his diaphragm up along his sternum. We did this primarily by bringing his felt awareness to the patterns of muscular tension. At times amplifying the muscular patterns brought more clarity to their contours. Purposefully embodying the muscular patterns helped him get more of a feel for who he was there. We explored the meaning from the bottom up by exploring what more *his body* knew about that posture and what it was expressing. He discovered that this pattern of muscular holding and tension expressed his discomfort with the prospect of initiating conversation between us. Initiating the conversation felt foreign. He discovered that the muscular pattern embodied how to pull back to avoid being seen. Over time, exploration of this holding pattern revealed a deep layer of frozen fear coupled with the crippling sense of not feeling good enough or important enough. He realized how this feeling had dogged him for a very long time. While this complex had significant familial aspects, it was rooted in the transgenerational predominance of cultural forces that had held a tenacious grip within his body, tragically obscuring the value of his heritage and somatic legacy.

Jackson had a keen proprioceptive sense. Proprioception is the sense of knowing where one is; where one's body is in physical space. Within the microcosm of the analytic vessel, he worked with and began to integrate the feeling that his unique voice mattered. One day, in a tender exploration between us, he found himself quite literally vibrating with aliveness. Moved deeply by his openness and vulnerability, I gently encouraged him to take it slowly, to stay with the experience of the vibrations, and notice what happened next inside—what sensations he became aware of. He spoke of a trembling vibration in his heart. He felt it both as quiet and yet big. His arms flushed with coolness, then heat and tingling. Tears pooled in his eyes. Slowly, words came, and he spoke of feeling connected to an energy all around him and between us. He felt the strength of his muscles right along with a soft tremulousness throughout. From this expanded, numinous state, he felt, for the first time, that he belonged; he had a place in this world. His proprioceptive sense of knowing where he was in space gained a psycho-spiritual dimension. He felt himself part of the natural order of things, a feeling of having a right to be on this earth (Fiori, David & Aglioti, 2014; Seth, 2013; Seth, Suzuki & Critchley, 2011; Baker, 2021).

Not unlike many people for whom the process of psychotherapy feels peculiarly alien, it proved more comfortable in the early stages of our work to explore his bodily experience than to pursue a more verbal inquiry alone (MacDonald, 2007).

Being with his bodily experience provided us with an entryway to his inner world. It cut through some of the psychological barriers that seemed so thick between us at the beginning of our work together that one could cut them with a knife. As the tensions eased a bit, we could talk more about that atmospheric pressure that had lain between us when we began. Exploring through a somatic vector grounded him in a territory of personal knowledge that was familiar, real, and immediate. Staying with the felt sense of his body gave him a foundation to venture further into his feelings. It served as an inner place to ground as we navigated his vulnerability. It brought a newfound awareness of his interiority and the discovery that he could share his inner world with another.

In contrast, my early attempts to work with him in a more traditional approach, based on verbal exploration, with its implicit bias based on the Western separation of body and mind, in which I did not address the embodied manifestations of his struggles and conflicts, shackled our process of analytic inquiry. Looking back, I can see how my countertransferential discomfort and fear propelled me in that direction at the start of our work, which transpired nearly 30 years ago. During my studies toward a master's degree in social work at New York University, I received extensive training on recognizing racism and institutional racism. However, the past five years have brought about even greater awareness of the depths of racism. Throughout this time, I have recognized more about my own racial biases and how they live at an implicit level in my body. Looking back, I wish I had been more nuanced and open to discussing the complex racial dynamics between Jackson and myself. I would have shared with him how I, too, had felt a kind of inner bracing when we commenced our work. I came to realize it stemmed more from the fact that he was a black man than my actual experience of him. I would have shared how this had troubled me as it was incongruent with my experience of him. In actuality, I did not feel any need to protect myself from him. I was protecting myself from a phantom narrative, a projection transmitted to me through generations (Kimbels, 2014). Such a dialogue, I think, would have created more mutuality and would have opened room for more to be explored, known, and felt.

Resmaa Menakem, author of *My Grandmother's Hands*, knows well how racialized trauma reverberates through our individual, relational, and transgenerational bodies. He brings the voice of Ta-Nehisi Coates to vivify this:

> But all our phrasing—race relations, racial chasm, racial injustice, racial profiling, white privilege, even white supremacy—serves to obscure that racism is a visceral experience, that it dislodges brains, blocks airways, rips muscle, extracts organs, cracks bones, breaks teeth ... You must always remember that the sociology, the history, the economics, the graphs, the charts, the regressions all land, with great violence, upon the body.
>
> (Ta-Nehisi Coates in Menakem, 2017, p. x)

Reflections on the Relevance of Intero- and Exteroceptive Awareness in Early Stages of Psychotherapeutic Work

When, in an attempt to guard against the insidious pain of transgenerational and culturally embedded racism, whether in the body of the therapist or of the patient, loosening that constraint in a relationally embodied psychotherapeutic process may offer hope. First, hope is engendered when psychotherapists, whether white or persons of color, recognize how the power dynamics inherent in the therapeutic situation might echo with residual dynamics intrinsic to slavery and racism, bringing consciousness to the potential of reenactment of these dynamics. Secondly, hope is engendered when through that collaboration, a psychic space is created such that each member of the dyad is able to settle within their bodily self and feel that within-ness as home, a home of which each individual has distinct ownership. Thirdly, hope lies in the possibility that two persons with differently colored bodies can find their way to consciously relate, with a relative sense of ease, in the same room, in the community of humanity. Exploration of interoceptive and exteroceptive awareness anchors affective intrapsychic experience in brain–body functioning, creating a non-shaming way into some of the most private subjective and intersubjective realms of psychic life, including implicit racial bias (MacDonald, 2007). Though I think more was possible in my work with Jackson, I know we were both touched and changed through our time together.

When the feeling of being alive has been shattered by terror, leaving a person no place to "be" and no place of safety to *body* into, as in the case of Eva, I believe the work of psychotherapy must include the body and the development of interoceptive awareness. There has to be a body for a psyche to dwell in; that is, there has to be some awareness of one's body for one to feel to be one's self, for one to feel to be an intact person (Winnicott, 1960).

Everything so many of us love about life unfolds in our body—sensing, seeing, feeling, and connecting with each other and the world. For many of us, this time of COVID-19 has highlighted a feel for just how important this is after having experienced for over two years the absence of "in-person" interaction. Seeing loved ones on the screen is not the same as being with another, "in-person," with their unique ways of moving about a space, movements as unique as a signature, that express the quality of a person's character. We might not even be conscious of knowing these movements until we realize we recognize that person amongst 50 others in a distant crowd because of their unique movement signature. Psychological isolation amplifies when our everyday tasks are devoid of "in-person" or in-bodied contact with others. The commercial world that seems able to capitalize on almost anything seems to want to seduce us into the insinuated benefit and glamour of a "touchless" world. Yet, we know that hearing a concert on Zoom is not the same as being with others listening to musicians make music, and feeling that bodily, skin-*tingling* resonance, that unique, almost magical feeling that can arise from hearing live music together with others—that feeling of being alive.

Prana—the Subtle Vibratory Aliveness of Your Body: A Meditation[5]

While remarkable, measuring interoception scientifically can induce a trance of narrowed perspective. By its very nature, science is at once highly complex yet limited. Science tends to separate in order to discern. In the case of measuring neuroception, while the felt experience of one's heartbeat signals the capacity to experience neuroception, it is essential to remember that multiple systems comprise the neuroceptive domain and, together, they are utterly more complex than one's heartbeat. This integral complexity interacts with exteroception and simultaneously with all life in a web of interdependence. The alchemist grasped something of that reality in the fundament of "as above so below."

A Meditation:

Interoception meets and integrates with exteroception—the hum of aliveness within—our natural birthright, the feeling of being alive. It is echoed in the whirling vastness one can hear when one quietens within and listens to what is outside at, for example, high altitudes in mountain wilderness. At that altitude, it is as though you can hear the earth spinning on its axis in relation to the cosmos—the earth in relation to the cosmos as the ego-self axis is within oneself. That link, though it can be impacted by humans, is of a magnitude beyond conceptual knowing. You can sense it, though Western culture does not emphasize such sensorial awareness. Yet if you go outside in the quiet of the night or at predawn, you can hear it when you quiet yourself.

If you are moved to, you might try it. Go outside in the quiet of the night or at predawn, and quiet yourself—quiet your body, perhaps through several full inhalations and exhalations.

As you exhale, bring your awareness to the path of your exhalation as it moves out and down your body. Notice the felt sense of the exhalation as it travels along its path. See if you can notice the letting go of the tension that is made possible in the process of exhalation. As you focus your attention on your felt sensation, notice how and to what extent your thoughts quiet.

Now listen to that which is outside of you.

If you are near unpaved patches of earth, you may, if you tune your listening, hear a hum that rises several inches from the floor of the earth and envelopes the earth—something like a sound aura. This is the sound of life rising from the earth's surface, be it your yard or a park or little patch of earth around a tree in the city.

Or if you are in a less urban area, listen to the desert floor, or the soft, thick floor of Arctic forests, or the vast open plains and chaparral, or perhaps a wetlands or other body of water.

Listen for the hum of insects, microbes, fungi, plants, and other little creatures, singing the world alive.

See if you can feel the pulsing of your heart as your veins spread across your body like the vast networks of watersheds traversing and nourishing the earth. You may have seen those veins of Earth from an airplane. Those waterways are the earth's lifeblood, just as is the blood pulsing through your heart and body.

The blissful hum of aliveness, or what is known in Sanskrit as *prana*, can be sensed as the telluric currents that invisibly guide the migratory movements of all the earth's creatures, which are also alive in your body, here, in this moment.

As you sense this hum of energy lying just below yet also within the physical surfaces of your body, you might notice a subtle but sure feeling of bliss. Not the euphoria that surges and ebbs but the ongoing stream of life that can be felt as happiness for no reason, what the Tantrics called *prana*.

Notes

1 Damasio (2021) perceives consciousness to be that which abides in organisms with nervous systems that interact with the aims of homeostasis. This is what gives rise to ownership of self-experience: subjectivity. While he bows to the remarkable intelligence and sensorial responsiveness of plants, bacteria, etc., because they lack nervous systems, which are the basis of self-reflection, he does not regard them as conscious.

    Fuchs (2018), on the other hand, addresses the question of consciousness from a phenomenological perspective, though not with disregard to neuroscience: "[L]ife always proceeds consciousness. It manifests itself primarily in a basic sense of the 'deep body' as the source and origin of conscious experience, not as its object."

2 A "*koan*" is a paradoxical anecdote or riddle without a solution, used in Zen Buddhism to demonstrate the inadequacy of logical reasoning and provoke enlightenment.

3 Authentic Movement, also known as Movement in Depth, has roots in Jungian Active Imagination. I will describe it at length in Chapter 9.

4 See my article, "Psyche within the Matrix of the Natural World: Weaving the Inner and Outer" https://onlinelibrary.wiley.com/share/author/6FUTSPVGEINIDC6WZMRK? target=10.1111/1468–5922.12874, https://doi.org/10.1111/1468–5922.12874

5 See Willa Blythe Baker (2021) for descriptions of and meditations on *prana*.

References

Avery, J. A., Drevets, W. C., Moseman, S. E., Bodurka, J., Barcalow, J. C., & Simmons, W. K. (2014). Major depressive disorder is associated with abnormal interoceptive activity and functional connectivity in the insula. *Biological Psychiatry, 76*(3), 258–266.

Baker, W. B. (2021). *The wakeful body: Somatic mindfulness as a path to freedom*. Boulder, CO: Shambala Publications.

Bernston, G. G., Gianaros, P. J., & Tsakiris, M. (2019). Interoception and the autonomic nervous system: Bottom-up meets top-down. In M. Tsakiris & H. De Preester (Eds.), *The interoceptive mind: From homeostasis to awareness*. Oxford: Oxford University Press.

Bright, B. (2010). Facing Medusa: Alchemical transformation through the power of surrender. Presented at the "Aesthetic Nature of Change" conference of the Institute for Cultural Change in Ojai, CA, May 22, 2010.

Cambray, J. (2012/2009). *Synchronicity: Nature and psyche in an interconnected universe*. Carolyn and Ernest Fay Series in Analytical Psychology, vol. 15., D. H. Rosen (series Ed.), College Station: Texas A&M University Press.

Chodorow, J. (1999). Dance therapy and the transcendent function. In P. Pallaro (Ed.), *Authentic movement: Essays by Mary Starks Whitehouse, Janet Adler and Joan Chodorow*. Philadelphia, PA: Kingsley.

Damasio, A. R. (1995). On some functions of the human prefrontal cortex. In J. Grafman, K. J. Holyoak, & F. Boller (Eds.), *Structure and functions of the human prefrontal cortex* (pp. 241–251). New York: New York Academy of Sciences.

—— (1999). *The feeling of what happens: Body and emotion in the making of consciousness*. New York: Harcourt Brace & Co.

—— (2021). *Feeling and knowing: Making minds conscious*. New York: Pantheon Books, a division of Random House.

Davies, J. M. (2022). Discussion of David Levit's "Somatic Experiencing." *Psychoanalytic Dialogues, 32*(3), 253–260. https://doi.org/10.1080/10481885.2022.2061157

—— (2023). Reawakening desire: Shame, mourning, analytic love, and psychoanalytic imagination. *Psychoanalytic Dialogues, 33*(3), 285–301. https://doi.org/10.1080/10481885.2023.2204773

Davies, J. M., & Frawley, M. G. (1994). *Treating the adult survivor of childhood sexual abuse: A psychoanalytic perspective*. New York: Basic Books.

Driscoll, R. (2020). *The sensing body in the visual arts: Making and experiencing sculpture*. London, New York: Bloomsbury Visual Arts.

Fiori, F., David, N., & Aglioti, S. M. (2014). Processing of proprioceptive and vestibular body signals and self-transcendence in Ashtanga yoga practitioners. *Frontiers in Human Neuroscience, 8*. https://doi.org/10.3389/fnhum.2014.00734

Fuchs, T. (2018). *Ecology of the brain*. Oxford: Oxford University Press.

—— (2020). The circularity of the embodied mind. *Frontiers in Psychology, 11*. https://doi.org/10.3389/fpsyg.2020.01707

Geurts, K. (2005). Consciousness as feeling in the body: A West African theory of embodiment, emotion and the making of mind. In D. Howes (Ed.), *Empire of the senses: The sensual culture reader* (pp. 164–178). Oxford: Berg.

Holifield, B. (2022). Psyche within the matrix of the natural world: Weaving the inner and outer. *Journal of Analytical Psychology, 67*(5), 1410–1430. https://doi.org/10.1111/1468-5922.12874

Howes, D. (Ed). (1991). *The varieties of sensory experience: A sourcebook in the anthropology of the senses*. Toronto: University of Toronto Press.

Joshi, V., Graziani, P., & Del-Monte, J. (2021). The role of interoceptive attention and appraisal in interoceptive regulation. *Frontiers in Psychology, 12*, 714641. https://doi.org/10.3389/fpsyg.2021.714641

Kalsched, D. (1996). *The Inner World of Trauma: Archetypal Defenses of the Personal Spirit*. London, New York: Routledge.

—— (2013). *Trauma and the soul: A psycho-spiritual approach to human development and its interruption.* New York: Routledge.

—— (2020). Opening the closed heart: Affect-focused work with victims of early trauma. *The Journal of Analytic Psychology, 65*(1), 136–152.

Kimbels, S. (2014) *Phantom narratives: The unseen contributions of culture to psyche.* Lanham, MD: Rowman & Littlefield.

Levine, P. A. (2010). *In an unspoken voice: How the body releases trauma and restores goodness.* Berkeley, CA: North Atlantic Books.

MacDonald, K. (2007). Interoceptive cues: When "gut feelings" point to anxiety. Current Psychiatry, 6(11), 49–62.

May, L. M., Kosek, P., Zeidan, F., & Berkman, E. T. (2014). The role of interoception in addiction: a critical review. Neuroscience and Biobehavioral Reviews, 36(8), 1857–1869.

Menakem, R. (2017*). In my grandmother's hands: Racialized trauma and the pathway to mending our hearts and bodies.* Las Vegas, NE: Central Recovery Press.

Pallaro, P. (Ed.). (1999). *Authentic movement: Essays by Mary Stark Whitehouse, Janet Adler and Joan Chodorow.* Philadelphia, PA & London: Jessica Kingsley.

Paulus, M. P., & Stein, M. B. (2010). Interoception in anxiety and depression. Brain Structure and Function, 214(5–6), 451–463.

Panksepp, J. (1998a). *Affective neuroscience: The foundations of human and animal emotions.* New York: Oxford University Press.

—— (1998b). The preconscious substrates of consciousness: Affective states and the evolutionary origins of the self. *Journal of Consciousness Studies, 5*(5–6), 566–582.

Payne, P., Levine, P. A., & Crane-Godreau, M. A. (2015). Somatic experiencing: Using interoception and proprioception as core elements of trauma therapy. *Frontiers in Psychology, 6*(93). https://doi.org/10.3389/fpsyg.2015.00093

Porges, S. (2019). Rethinking trauma: Polyvagal theory can revolutionize your work with trauma survivors. An interview with Ruth Buczynski at the National Institute for the Clinical Application of Behavioral Medicine. https://s3.amazonaws.com/nicabm-stealthseminar/Rethinking-trauma-new/Stephen/NICABM-StephenPorges_Part5-Transcript.pdf

Racker, H. (1957). The meanings and uses of countertransference. The Psychoanalytic Quarterly, 26, 303–357.

Scarry, E. (1985). *The body in pain.* New York: Oxford University Press.

Schore, A. N. (2009). Right-brain affect regulation: An essential mechanism of development, trauma, dissociation, and psychotherapy. In D. Fosha, D. Siegel, & M. Solomon (Eds.), *The healing power of emotion: Affective neuroscience, development & clinical practice* (Norton Series on Interpersonal Neurobiology). New York: W. W. Norton.

—— (2011). The right brain implicit self lies at the core of psychoanalysis. Psychoanalytic Dialogues, 21(1), 75–100.

Sedeño, L., Couto, B., Melloni, M., Canales-Johnson, A., Yoris, A., Baez, S., Esteves, S., Velásquez, M., Barttfeld, P., Sigman, M., Kichic, R., Chialvo, D., Manes, F., Bekinschtein, T. A., & Ibanez, A. (2014). How do you feel when you can't feel your body? Interoception, functional connectivity and emotional processing in depersonalization-derealization disorder. *PLoS ONE, 9*(6). https://doi.org/10.1371/journal.pone.0098769

Seth, A. K. (2013). Interoceptive inference, emotion, and the embodied self. *Trends Cognitive Science, 17*, 565–573. https://doi.org/10.1016/j.tics.2013.09.007

Seth, A. K., Suzuki, K., & Critchley, H. D. (2011). An interoceptive predictive coding model of conscious presence. *Frontiers in Psychology, 2*, 395. https://doi.org/10.3389/fpsyg.2011.00395

Siegel, D. J. (2007). *The mindful brain: Reflection and attunement in the cultivation of well-being*. New York: W. W. Norton.

Soth, M. (2019). The relational turn in body psychotherapy. In *The Routledge international handbook of embodied perspectives in psychotherapy*. London, New York: Routledge.

Stern, D. B. (2019). *The infinity of the unsaid: Unformulated experience, language, and the nonverbal*. New York: Routledge.

Stern, D. N. (1985). *The interpersonal world of the infant*. New York: Basic Books.

Tronick, E. Z., Heidelise, A., Adamson, L., Wise, S., & Brazelton, T. B. (1978). The infant's response to entrapment between contradictory messages in face-to-face interaction. *Journal of the American Academy of Child Psychiatry, 17*(1), 1–13.

Winnicott, D. W. (1960). The theory of the parent–infant relationship. *International Journal of Psycho-Analysis, 41*, 585–595.

Woodman, M. (1987). An interview with Marion Woodman. *Parabola, 12*(2), 4. https://parabola.org/2019/04/13/worshipping-illusions-an-interview-with-marion-woodman/

Chapter 3

Body-Based Inquiries

Staying with the theme of the Linda Hogan poem *There Are Many Ways In*, which opens this book, in this chapter I will describe a few ways one might evoke bodily-based awareness. These may be useful for the therapist exploring their own somatic unconscious, and in their work with patients. I think of these ways of evoking body-based awareness as guiding principles rather than techniques or a particular methodology. They will always need to be rooted in the lived moment, which will give the manner of communication its own shape and quality. For me, inviting another to bring awareness to their bodily experience inevitably deepens my own and, thus, the distinct relational experience between us. Jung emphasizes the necessity of the body in achieving differentiation, whether inter- or intrapsychic:

> And really, the essence of differentiation, the idea of the Self, could not exist for one moment if there were not a body to create and maintain that distinctness. We may suppose that if the body vanishes and disintegrates, the Self in a way disintegrates, for it loses its confines.
>
> (Jung, 1934, p. 236)

Attention

Foremost, of course, is the therapist's awareness of their own bodily-based sense of self. The most valuable tool to attain this awareness is generous interest in and attention to immediate experience. Freud put forth that psychoanalysts must each participate in their own psychoanalysis. The reason was not so much weighted on the analyst being fully analyzed as it was on the analyst, through their own experience of analysis, fully recognizing the existence of the unconscious, "the presence within us of this paradoxical (strange but familiar) self … the one we have learned about in our own analysis and elsewhere" (Grotstein, 2000, p. 113). In parallel, the therapist's awareness of the dimensionality of their own bodily existence will serve as their most valuable resource.

Perhaps the simplest and potentially the most profound of inquiries is to bring attention to the breath just as it is, without trying to change it. Inevitably, the

DOI: 10.4324/9781003305804-4

breathing pattern will shift and adjust. This self-regulating function is initiated simply by one's attention. Sustained attention to this new breathing pattern furthers and deepens the self-regulation process. One could allow one's breath to serve as a light, alerting you to sensations—those that are foreground as well as those that are faint or more like a sense of an absence of sensation. Staying with these inward places, curious about the felt sensation of what is happening, and being attentive to what happens next is the practice, whether it be an intensification of the sensation, awareness of an affect, an image, a movement (the most subtle, near imperceptible, like a change in heartbeat or a rigidification around one's bones or a simple postural adjustment or an expressive gesture).

The body is, at times, the ego; at times, the unconscious; and, at times, the bridge between the two. However, it is not enough to know or conceptualize this formulation; one has to feel it. The tendency to conceive of body as separate from mind is rooted in cultural and familial attitudes as well as psychological insults, injuries, and trauma. Transcending this polarization requires intent and practice. Ideally, the psychotherapist participates in some form of psychotherapeutic process that incorporates the somatic dimension of the psyche. However, it can also be approached through one's daily contemplative practices, in which one purposely brings attention to the felt sense of breathing, sensing, walking, sitting, and moving.

Additionally, it is essential for the psychotherapist to cultivate awareness of how what we usually ascribe to bodily life is linked to what we ascribe to emotional life. In other words, to purposefully bring attention to the bodily-felt sense of emotions and how we defend against them. Bringing awareness to the bodily-felt quality of highly nuanced states of psychic life is equally important.

Patience

Patience is surely a needed attribute. Life in the body is a moment-to-moment unfolding. The body has a different pace than thinking or intuition. While attention itself has a powerful effect on bringing consciousness to the bodily basis of experience, patience is required to linger in an attuned way to the unfolding experience. Once attention is brought to the felt experience of breathing and sensations, one enters the river of life's unfolding, where each moment is new. Emotion gains substantive dimensionality, like carefully peering into deep, clear water in contrast to seeing only the water's surface qualities.

The patience required of being with, and not knowing what will come from attending to bodily-based experience, is similar in kind, though perhaps directed to a different domain, as that which Bion refers to when he eloquently implores us to listen without memory or desire (Bion, 1988).[1] Perhaps most significant within the psychotherapy culture is to refrain from interpretation and meaning-making, which can all too quickly foreclose on the *hidden body*, the body that wants to be known but also may not. Direct bodily-based experience does not ruminate on the past or anticipate the future. It unfolds in a radical now (Baker, 2021).

Opening

Many years ago, I had the opportunity to work with a very unusual man, Oscar Aguado, in a contemplative movement practice that I would describe as falling somewhere between dance and Tai Chi. "The Form," which is what he called the practice, is a meditation in moving, in which one's intention is dedicated to finding the circularity within musculoskeletal alignment and the flow state this induces. Moving in this way, though full of muscular engagement, feels effortless. This had the effect of putting me into something like a state of grace. I do not think the felt experience I found in effortfully effortless movement will ever leave me. While I only rarely achieve such a state, the memory lives in my cells, and that background awareness informs me. Some of his guiding phrases stay with me, such as: "Make love to the ground as you walk." He also used more off-handed correctives when referencing one's muscular patterns manifest in mundane tasks: "You are brushing your teeth, and you are killing yourself!" What he meant to bring attention to is how much more "open" we can be than we are typically aware of. Willa Blythe Baker, who teaches Tibetan Buddhism as a path of awakening through the body, describes how when one opens one's body and senses, "you notice energy flowing throughout your body and flowing between your body and the outside world" (2021, p. 109). She speaks of this as the subtle body that abides in what we tend to think of as our physical form. She calls on us to

> Notice the vibrant wakeful quality of your body's energy field. When you find yourself closing down into a narrow perception of anything, offer yourself this simple instruction: "Open." ... Let your body be a support for opening up to the world, your sense experiences, and your inner landscape.
>
> (Baker 2021, p. 109)

Entering the Sensory Experience of Each Moment

In a similar vein, Charlotte Selver, the founder of the practice known as Sensory Awareness, would frequently encourage inquiries such as:

> Are you open for this possibility of the energy source of breathing to go through you or are you collapsing? Are you open to this coming and going of air and the possibility—whether we sit, or stand, or lie—to allow this exchange of air through us?
>
> (Selver, 1985, speaking at a conference at Esalen Institute)

Each of these inquiries can be an invaluable way for a therapist to evoke awareness of their own bodily selves more fully. As psychotherapists, we can make a practice of such simple inquiries. As we ground ourselves in our own knowing, we can pursue inquiry with those with whom we work in an attuned and empathic manner. We might continue to inquire of ourselves and our patients, "Is your breath there for the sadness you feel?" Staying oriented to the fact that sensation is the bodily basis of emotion, we could take the inquiry further, into whether the patient senses that their breath is there, or whether the question prompts them to breathe, or whether it brings their awareness to the fact that their breath is not supportive of feeling but is actually an active aspect of protecting against feeling. We might simply ask, "What is that like inside?" A valuable next step that can aid in staying with the moment-to-moment bodily-based unfolding could be something as simple as, "Stay with the felt sensations and notice what sensation comes into your awareness next." In this manner, the therapist cleaves to tracking bodily sensations.

A more open-ended inquiry is, "What happens next; maybe you notice other sensations or perhaps a feeling, an image, or maybe a memory?" This inquiry makes room for affect, image, or memory. However, the danger is that of overriding the body. Not leaving room for other forms of awareness may feel contrived, narrow a patient's attention, or even foreclose on affect. As genuine feelings arise, the therapist can maintain attentiveness to the patient's link to the bodily basis of these experiences, especially when engaging implicit memory, because much of what is not known to the conscious mind is held in the body. As affect arises that has previously been defended against, those defensive structures, which have their own bodily basis, might reemerge quickly. Staying with the bodily basis of the defensive structures can be a very helpful way to avoid getting bogged down in what Jung called a psychological complex. Sometimes, moving back and forth between the somatic basis of the familiar defense and the new experience is a refreshing way to let the new experience psychophysically imprint. New awareness, affect, and insight must be grounded—felt in the body—to be thoroughly integrated.

When a patient moves out of sensorial experience and into a different domain, I might backstitch, gently asking, "What sensations are you aware of now?" for example, or, "Oh, yeah, feeling hurt; where do you feel that in your body? What sensations do you notice there? What (sensations) happen next?" If an image or memory arises, I will likely encourage slowing down and I might ask something like, "What is the felt sense in your body of that image? Alternatively, bring the image into your body, stay there with it a bit, and notice the felt sense in your body."

As you can see, the inquiries are very simple. The genuine attunement that arises from one's own embodied knowing brings them alive. The main point is staying with what we most likely otherwise pass over, the somatic basis of experience, and how doing so can deepen the psyche's unfolding.

From a psychoneurological perspective, implicit memory is primarily correlated with activity on the right side of the brain, which is also the area of the brain associated with imagination, dreams, and affect (Schore, 2019). Not infrequently, in the exploration of somatic experience, a dream suddenly comes to consciousness, which I most always make room for while sensitively continuing to stay oriented to the unfolding bodily states, affects, and associations. Dreams lace the somatic basis of exploration with the mythopoetic meaning that carries the soul. Incorporating attention to the felt experience in the body can allow affects to be more fully known. In *Memories, Dreams, and Reflections*, Jung (1965/1961) spoke of how finding the images concealed in the emotions was inwardly reassuring and calming. Bringing attention to the sensorial felt experience of affect brings an added dimension. It furthers the calming effect when needed and brings awareness to the deadening or withdrawal of sensation from affects that are hard to bear. As the capacity to tolerate affects deepens and emotions begin to formulate, the accompanying images felt in and through the body enrich the unfolding psychic process.

Working with Bodily-felt Pain

In the Chapter 2 vignette of Jackson, I described how we worked on addressing his experience of pain. Doing so became a way into his inner world, and offered a way to access his feelings. When someone expresses feeling bodily pain and exploring it might open more dimensionality of the inner world, there are many options.

Most of us instinctually want to get rid of, or move away from, pain. Here, the intention is to be with it; in so doing, it may amplify, dissipate, morph, or potentially psychophysically flood the patient. Sometimes, bringing gentle, felt attention to a painful area in the body does allow the pain to melt. Here, attention acts a bit like the sun on ice, with the warmth of attention melting the ice into water. Water, like emotion, is more fluid and constantly changing. Naming emotion and exploring it, as we know, can facilitate psychic process. Insight might arise quickly, and the patient is back on track. Alternatively, it may become the territory that the therapeutic couple explores over time. Often, pain needs sustained attention.

Bringing attention to pain's shape, contour, and color is a beginning. Eliciting a detailed description of its action can be useful, e.g., if the pain has been described as a tight rope, one could inquire further and perhaps offer options such as, "Does the rope twist in toward your spine or pull outward in a taught strain?" One might also explore the function by simply asking, "What is the function of the pull?" Sometimes, if the pain seems uncontactable, as if located somewhere in a dense fog, I might inquire about the space around it (as an example). "Just notice the space above and below that dark, heavy ball in your solar plexus; what is it like? What if you just let yourself feel the quality of the space around the dark density of the ball? Notice what happens next."

If, for instance, a patient reports that their heart is beating uncomfortably fast and exploring it in the manner above has not brought about any significant shift, I might ask, "What if you expressed through a gesture in your hands what it feels like in your heart?" I might follow with, "Try expressing, with your hands, what you would like to feel" (Mindell, 1982). This often is surprising, bringing the patient a sense of agency versus helplessness. Further inquiry can then unfold. Though shifts in the experience of pain or tension do occur as we bring attention to them, it is necessary to begin by accepting the feeling as it is. Otherwise, the pain is likely to become mercurial, doubling down, darting here and there.

Amplification and Matching

The existential meaning in postures, facial expressions, tensional patterns, and gestures can all be explored by purposely entering the felt sensation and overall felt sense of the posture. Inviting awareness into the felt experience can reveal what verbal expressions override. The exploration can be furthered by staying with it, with inquiries such as, "What more does your body know about that?" Physically amplifying the postural or tensional expression, subtly at first, then furthering the amplification until recognition overrides unconscious action, can bring more learning. From there, many possible ways to further discover what is being expressed can follow through inquiries such as:

- "What wants to happen?"
- "Is there a gesture, sound, or movement?"
- "What is the function of the pattern?"
- "Are there words or a phrase that arises?"
- "What does your body know it needs?"

These inquiries are directed toward the implicit or procedural self's way of knowing rather than the verbal self's conceptual meaning.

A patient of mine who had witnessed a great deal of violence when young often felt tension around her eyes and solar plexus. Exploration revealed the part of her that would get sleepy and "did not want to see" (dissociate). The pattern of tightening the solar plexus was discovered to be an attempt to both disappear and withdraw so as not to be seen or attacked and, ultimately, not to inhale so as not to feel (deny or dissociate).

Once awareness is gleaned by doing the action "on purpose"[2] rather than out of one's awareness, it can be very useful to let it go "on purpose" by feeling the pathway of release through and out of the body. It can be of great value to bring conscious felt awareness to the gestalt of experience in the released state, allowing for the new experience to imprint in the body–mind and for insight and affect to be known and shared.

Turning Inward Sensing the Feeling Body

Turning inward drop down from your thinking mind toward the felt sense of your body. Direct your inward attention toward restless or stagnant energies and notice where you experience them in your body. Perhaps emotion is quite prevalent, igniting rumination or running thoughts such that you are unaware of your body. Perhaps you experience constriction in your abdomen and tensional holding in your chest, shoulders, eyes, head, or jaw. Perhaps you feel stress all over, like static on a screen. Perhaps you feel "down" or "dulled"—shoulders pulling in and chest weighted—or an atmospheric inner/outer numbness. As the analyst or the analytic couple brings joint attention to these internal territories, there is a sense of having descended into the psycho-physical realm. By closely attending, something inside might begin to open up.

Subtle Energies of the Nervous System

In Psychotherapeutic Process

As psychotherapists, we focus on regulating states of hyper- and hypo-arousal of the nervous system to bring about enough quieting or quickening so that emotions having their basis in those states can be brought to consciousness. Developing tolerance of sensation deepens affect tolerance. Emotions can then be more fully borne and symbolized. With the upsurge in psychoneurological discoveries, it is common to hear remarks like: "My nervous system cannot handle it," "I am stuck in my reptilian brain," or "I am all about fight–flight." While these off-handed remarks likely point to actual experience, people all too often get caught in that "place," in other words, resigned to the inner state they find themselves in. The work of psychotherapy that includes the somatic dimension is to recognize and pursue an inquiry into the bodily-felt dynamic. Restorative gestures, images, dreams, memories, attitudes, or catalytic relational interactions may arise in the process of resolution to the tensional cycle. By employing analytic discipline and not jumping ahead of the body's pacing, psychological processing unfolds from the bottom up, allowing meaning to emerge (Schore, 2003; Ogden, Minton & Paine, 2006; Siegel, 2006). When this occurs, the analytic space opens, and generative exploration resumes. Both in the dyad find relief from psychophysical constriction; perhaps breathing becomes more synchronous between the two, and sometimes there is an opening of the closed heart (Kalsched, 2020).

Transformative Practices

For centuries, spiritual traditions have cultivated the energies that run the length of the spinal column—understandably, as it is that which gives structure; it scaffolds the strength and flexibility of our organism, aptly referred to in some traditions as the cosmic ladder or cosmic tree, connecting us to earth and sky. The spinal column houses the spinal cord, the aspect of the brain situated in the core of the body. Branches and tendrils of nerves expand out from that central cord, electric with energy, interacting with organs, limbs, fingers, toes, and skin. If the blood that flows through our veins can be likened to the waterways that course the earth, then the nervous system can be likened to the earth's telluric currents and electromagnetic field. Our neural system receives and transmits information through a constant looping process, moving from inside the body out and outside the body in. It is alive and electric. In many traditions, this vertical column is imagined as a conduit of powerful, subtle energy. It is known as the cosmic serpent, kundalini, the mother channel, the chakra channel, the Du Meridian, or Governing channel through which Qui flows in our body.

Willa Blythe Baker describes one of these, the mother channel, in detail, as extending from the crown of the head to the base of the spine. It is referred to in the feminine and known in Sanskrit as *uma*, "the mother in the center."

> The uma is subtle and straight, the color of a deep-blue summer sky. Like all pathways in the body, it is not solid. It is made of light, of energy.
>
> Somehow, the uma is locatable in the body, but its interior is an infinite expanse, like a cloudless sky. It is a paradox, having infinity in our core. We so often think of our body as a temporary home. Perhaps this is what makes mother-channel meditation so powerful. We experience humanness coexisting with transcendence.
>
> (Baker, 2021, p. 96)

In hearing the various ways this archetypal energy is imaged and named, you may find that one image piques your imagination more than others. A direct embodied experience can transform the archetypal image into an archetypal experience. To get a feel for this, when you have a quiet moment, perhaps before sleep or upon awakening, you might explore the following guided meditation on the mother channel:

> Close your eyes and imagine your body is made of energy and light like a vivid hologram.
>
> Now, drop down into the core of your body.
>
> Do not just witness the core. Flow down into your core with your consciousness so that you are inside your energy light body.
>
> There, extending from the crown of your head to the base of your spine is a column of light. As you enter the column of light, you encounter an open, endless sky right in the core of your body.
>
> Now, connect to the feeling of your breath.
>
> Breathing through your nostrils, gradually deepen your inhales and exhales.
>
> As you inhale, breathe into the sky-like mother channel in the core of your body.
>
> As you exhale, release the light and space of the mother channel on your out-breath so that it mixes with the space all around you.
>
> Long, slow, deep, gentle inhales. Long, slow, deep, gentle exhales.
>
> Continue for about five minutes.
>
> Then rest with your eyes open, heart open, mind open.
>
> (Baker, 2021, p. 96)

Baker further elucidates the meditation experience, noting that this pathway links the civilized with the sensual while also connecting our head with our heart and earth with heaven:

> The yogic texts say the mother channel is the place where enlightenment ultimately happens. It is where the restless energy winds gather and dissolve into

stillness. This is why connecting to its interior is important. Bringing attention to the mother channel in meditation and yoga can be a powerful way to connect to pure consciousness not as an idea but as a somatic experience.

(Baker, 2021, pp. 96–97)

When exploring the mother channel meditation, I find my imagination moving between the expansive blue sky and the extraordinary indigo-blue ocean waters of the Hawaiian Islands. Even while diving at great depths, the light somehow emanates from within the water itself. This gives me a feel for the unending depths and expanse of infinity. I find it profound to experience that the wounds and traumas that stir the restless energies in our nervous system are also the portals to transformative energies through which we expand beyond our familiar identities of ego and self into union with an infinite expanse of life.

Grotstein, whom I referenced at the beginning of this chapter, reflects on Freud's often-quoted statement, "Where id was there ego will be" (Freud, 1933), raising a question:

but must the id truly yield to the ego? Moreover, why does the id not have a more personal name than "it"? I am suggesting that the id is really the alter ego and that it expresses itself to us subjectively as the Ineffable Subject of Being.

(Grotstein, 2000, p. 113)

When Grotstein speaks of the unconscious as the Ineffable Subject of Being, it intersects with the numinosity that is a potential aspect of bodily existence. Here, one can sense and feel the body as it shape-shifts through the collective unconscious into the personal, the invisible existing within the visible. The substantive physical body is the container of all such unfolding. Grotstein puts it this way: "The ineffable Subject speaks to his Phenomenal subject, who feels—through sense (noticing), myth (unconscious phantasy), and passion (caring)—reflexively through the analyst container" (Grotstein, 2000, pp. 114–115).

I choose Grotstein because very few in the psychoanalytic community discuss how we work to gain the ability "to transcend our defensiveness … in order to become one with our *aliveness* (Ogden, 1997) or with our very being-ness, or Dasein" (Heidegger, 1927; Grotstein, 2000, p. 300). Embodying these states gives a felt dimensionality to the endeavor.

Notes

1 From Bion's *Notes on Memory and Desire* (1988), "with the operation of judgment psychoanalytic 'observation' is concerned neither with what has happened nor with what is going to happen but with what is happening."
2 See Behnke (1995) "Matching."

References

Baker, W. B. (2021). *The wakeful body: Somatic mindfulness as a path to freedom*. Boulder, CO: Shambala Publications.

Behnke, E. A. (1995). Matching. In D. H. Johnson (Ed.), *Bone, breath and gesture* (pp. 317–337). Berkeley, CA: North Atlantic Books, California Institute of Integral Studies.

Bion, W. R. (1988). Notes on memory and desire. In E. B. Spillius (Ed.), *Melanie Klein today: Developments in theory and practice, Vol. 2. Mainly practice* (pp. 17–21). London: Taylor & Frances/Routledge. (Notes first published in 1967 in *The Psychoanalytic Forum 2*: 272–273, 279–280).

Freud, S. (1933). *New introductory lectures on psycho-analysis*. New York: W. W. Norton.

Grotstein, J. S. (2000). *Who is the dreamer who dreams the dream*. Hillsdale, NJ: The Analytic Press.

Heidegger, M. (1927). *Being and time*. New York: HarperCollins.

Jung, C. G. (1965/1961). *Memories, dreams, and reflections*. New York: Vintage Books, A Division of Random House.

——— (1989/1934). In J. Jarrett (Ed.), *Nietzsche's Zarathustra: Notes of the seminar given in 1934–1939*. New York: Routledge.

Kalsched, D. (2020). Opening the closed heart: Affect-focused work with victims of early trauma. *The Journal of Analytic Psychology*, *65*(1), pp. 136–152.

Mindell, A. (1982). *Dreambody: The body's role in revealing the self*. Boston, MA: Sigo Press.

Ogden, P., Minton, K, & Pain, C. (2006). *Trauma and the body: A sensorimotor approach to psychotherapy*. New York: W. W. Norton.

Ogden, T. H. (1997). *Reverie and interpretation: Sensing something human*. London: Routledge.

Schore. A. N. (2003). *Affect regulation and repair of the self*. New York: W. W. Norton.

——— (2019). *Right brain psychotherapy* (Norton Series on Interpersonal Neurobiology). New York: W. W. Norton.

Selver, C. (1985). Retrieved October 28, 2022, from www.storemypic.com/album/charlotte-selver-quotes.PR1/?sort=date_asc&page=1, A personal communication at an Esalen Institute conference in 1985.

Siegel, D. J. (2006) Foreword. In P. Ogden, K. Minton, & C. Pain (Eds.), *Trauma and the body: A sensorimotor approach to psychotherapy*. New York: W. W. Norton.

Chapter 4

Attaining Embodiment

A Developmental Perspective

In my practice as a Jungian analyst, attentive to the somatic basis of experience, I always seek research and theoretical perspectives that illuminate the territory and further the understanding of what I see and feel unfold in clinical practice. While neuroscience offers one *way in* to think about what we feel, or sometimes do not feel, in our bodies, developmental theories provide another. "From the moment of emergence into this world and through much of the first year of our life, it is through the somatic dimension of experience that we come to know ourselves and the ones who relate and care for us" (Driscoll, 2020, pp. 3–4). Developmental trauma, particularly pervasive developmental trauma, can severely disrupt the foundations of an experiential sense of embodiment. This chapter considers the developmental theory of Daniel Stern, which is rooted in empirical findings of research with infants by him and others, as well as W. D. Winnicott's thoughts on indwelling. Together, these views offer a basis for understanding the developmental processes of attaining—or failing to attain—an experiential sense of embodiment.

Daniel Stern's research into infancy has contributed enormously to our understanding of the nonverbal, bodily realm of human experience. Unlike other developmental theorists, Stern includes the significance of the body in each step of human development. Like the image on the front cover of this book, we become a person from our very beginnings through palpable bodily interactions with another, without which humans cannot survive. Based on extensive research, Stern elucidates the formation of a sense of self as it unfolds within an *interpersonal matrix* (2018/1985). While the body is always primary in development, each domain he delineates, from emergence through the development of a core sense of self, a subjective sense of self, and onward to a verbal sense of self, contributes to an *experiential* sense of embodiment, or its disruption. While earlier psychoanalytic developmental models posited that the primary task of development is that of self/other differentiation, Stern's research with actual infants found the opposite: neonates are able to distinguish self from other at birth. His findings highlight how the development of self occurs *through the creation of ties* with the primary caretaker(s) and *increasing relatedness*.

Making it abundantly clear that neonates are able to distinguish a sense of self from the very beginning of life shifts the long-held developmental view

DOI: 10.4324/9781003305804-5

that conceptualizes phases of normal autism, primary narcissism, and symbiosis (Mahler& Furer, 1968).[1] By establishing that self and other differentiation co-occur through the establishment of healthy ties to the other, this research dispels earlier notions that the attainment of an autonomous sense of self is found through gradual separation from the other. Stern's research details how the processes of affect attunement are essential because they contribute to attachment security and the capacity for intimacy. It describes in detail the bodily basis of experience that is foundational to relationship (Beebe & Lachmann,1988; Stern, 2018).

The Significance of Implicit Memories in Psychotherapy

Until around nine to ten months of age, the infant lives in a nonverbal experience of self. The nonverbal foundations or implicit knowledge shaped in that time are integral aspects of interpersonal life that continue to be shaped and reshaped throughout the life cycle. Because of their profound significance, finding ways to access these bodily-based, preverbal attributes of experience can significantly augment the work of depth psychotherapy. While developmentalists and body-oriented therapists are comfortable dealing with nonverbal communication, "most psychoanalysts, however, are not; they are more at ease with words, narrative and meaning ... A sort of zone of turbulence exists where the verbal and nonverbal meet" (Stern, 2018, p. xii). Finding the implicit or organizing pattern of emotion in nonverbal realms helps bridge that gap. There is now a broad consensus that identifies the domain of implicit knowledge to be where the vast majority of therapeutic change occurs (Sander et al., 1998; Stern, 1998; Schore, 2009; Ogden, Minton & Pain, 2006).

Awareness arising from bodily-felt experience gives palpable structure to an experience of self, much like the foundation that warp threads create in weaving; those threads—like the body—are always present even if, more often than not, they are outside our awareness. In a weaving, the warp threads provide basic structure and lend interest to the woven work, allowing it to pop with color or hum with textural and visual nuance; it is similar to how a felt sense of the body, when made conscious, vivifies the nuances of the feeling of being alive.

The small interactive, repetitive patterns of self interacting with others that psychodynamic theorists formerly referred to as internal objects are not objects but representations of patterns of interactions with others. Stern (2018) prefers to term these internal patterns "ways-of-being-with" to elicit a more experience-near feeling of the inner phenomena. Reformulating this concept delimits how a subjective world can be constituted before attributing innate features of fantasies, preferences, values, and action tendencies. These patterns, which become part of implicit memory, can be made conscious in the microanalysis and exploration of here-and-now experiences in the body. This offers a generative way to facilitate experiential shifts in one's way of relating to self and others. In this way, bringing attention to the bodily basis of psychodynamics can be woven into other traditional approaches.

Infant research itself unfolds through microanalysis of moment-to-moment, mostly nonverbal experiences. Because these fine details of the infant's nonverbal world offer a view of the territory encountered when exploring the elements of experience that comprise the implicit memories of adults, I will review some of the more salient aspects here.

The Three Domains of the Preverbal Intersubjective Sense of Self

Stern's research (2018), along with that of Beebe & Lachmann (1988), Braten (1998), and Trevarthen (1979), posits that infants have the capacity for primary intersubjectivity at the beginning of life. Stern's research with infants led to the conception of development unfolding as domains of experience that interact and layer. Stern's most updated view, in 2018, is that there are three subcategories of the preverbal sense of self: the emergent sense of self, the physical or core sense of self, and the subjective (or secondary intersubjective) sense of self. Each "sense of self" pertains to a domain of experience. While he initially believed that each had a particularly sensitive development period in the preverbal infant, he later realized that all three emerged together. These subcategories describe the specific developmental capacities that unfold in the early stages of intersubjective life. By virtue of their dynamic interaction, each contributes to the other in the infant's development. Unlike other phase-specific developmental models, one domain of a sense of self *is not relinquished* as the other takes hold. While each domain of experience has a particularly sensitive stage in the infant's development, at any point in the life cycle (as well as in a single therapy hour), events may occur that are more situated within one domain than another (Stern, 2018). Domains of a sense of self thus continually shift in and out of the foreground, weaving depth and texture into the lived moment.

1.   *The Emergent Sense of Self*

An emergent sense of self is that domain whose particularly sensitive developmental time frame is from birth through the second month of life. As discussed in Chapter 2, neuroscience shows how infants are born with a basic self-affectivity. Stern furthers that premise, recognizing that aspect of the infant's self that is able to yoke various perceptions so as to experience an emerging sense of oneself as a whole distinct being and to grasp a distinct sense of an other (Stern, 1985, p. 60). The emergent sense of self is that part of self that sensorially experiences the feeling of being alive, encounters the world in the moment, and gleans the gestalt of self and others through this. Stern writes: "All learning and creative acts begin in the domain of emergent relatedness. That domain alone is concerned with the coming-into-being of organization that is at the heart of creating and learning (1985, p. 67).

  Stern's research makes it clear that infants are capable of basic self-awareness: discerning their body as distinct from the objects around them, their own bodily actions distinct from the movements of other people, a sense of self-agency when producing sounds that they hear and movements that they feel (1985). As discussed in Chapter 2, all conscious experience implies a pre-reflective self-awareness or self-affection (Zahavi, 1999).

Clinical theorists such as Michael Balint, Melanie Klein, Harry Stack Sullivan, Ronald Fairbairn, Ronald Guntrip, and Mary Ainsworth and other attachment theorists, also believed that human social relatedness was present from birth. While they identified some of the salient experiences of internal state fluctuations and social relatedness that could contribute to a sense of self, the developmentalists furthered these perceptions, discovering the bodily-based capacities that lead the infant to use these experiences to differentiate self and other.

1a.   The Emergent Sense of Self and the Primacy of the Body

The first reference point for the infant that contributes to having a sense of self concerns an *organized sense of their body* in terms of actions, feeling states, and memories. In the emergent phase of an infant's early sense of self, the focus is on learning the relations between sensory experiences. The emergent sense of self takes form based on apprehending relationships between isolated experiences and processes. Infants seem to have a remarkable capacity for amodal perception, that is, they can take information received in one sensory modality and somehow translate it into another sensory modality. For instance, an infant can *visually* discern a specific pacifier from other pacifiers, even when their previous experience of it was solely via their *mouth*. This is achieved via sensorial memory of the felt texture in the mouth that is later linked to its visual presentation.

This same capacity of integrating visual and tactile sensations, even in the absence of repeated experience, is present in newborn infants, who are able to sense the two breasts of the mother as an integrated, coherent sense of breasts that belong to their mother. This contrasts earlier formulations based on Piagetian and most psychoanalytic accounts, which conceive the infant perceiving one breast as completely unrelated to another.

> Research shows that actual infants do not need repeated experience to begin to form some of the aspects of an emergent self and other. They are pre-designed to forge certain integrations ... The amount of cross-modal fluency in terms of predesign is extraordinary.
>
> (Stern, 2018, pp. 50–51)

This includes proprioceptive and visual, as well as auditory and visual amodal integration as it pertains to shape, intensity level, motion, number, and rhythm. Additionally, aspects of people will be experienced and remembered via the perception of their (categorical) affects, such as happy, sad, anger, interest, or disgust (Werner, 1948). And yet another experience of people is discerned through what Stern calls vitality affects, meaning those affects that do not fit the existing lexicon of affects but are better captured by their inherent kinesthetic dynamic. For instance, choppy actions—the motion of an adult rising from their chair, the cadence of their voice, or way of holding the infant—can be organized by the infant into a quality that is yoked to a particular caretaker. In this way, the infant has an emergent sense of the other.

2.   The Sense of a Core or Physical Self

Stern found that the sensitive time for the developmental domain of the sense of core or physical self is from two to six months. Experience in this domain coheres to allow for core relatedness, which pertains to self-agency, self-coherence, and self-continuity in time. Self-affectivity is here, too, but is already primary in the emergent sense of self.

> A crucial term here is a "sense of," as distinct from "concept of" or "knowledge of" or "awareness of" a self or other. The emphasis is on the palpable experiential realities of substance, action, sensation, affect, and time. Sense of self is not a cognitive construct. It is an experiential integration. This sense of a core self will be the foundation for all the more elaborate senses of the self to be added on later.
>
> (Stern, 1985, p. 71)

2a.   The Sense of the Core Self with Other

Infants' response to the others' embodied affects can be seen in affectively synchronous dyadic interaction that emerges around two to three months (Trevarthen, 1979; Stern, 1985). These dyadic states of awareness arising from affect attunement, bodily resonance, and intercorporeality have been finely detailed via microanalysis of moment-to-moment interaction between mothers and babies (Beebe, Cohen & Lachmann, 2016). They documented, via video and drawings, infants' and parents' interactions at four months (https://youtu.be/TifkQl3iOdc). They show how the faces of infants and parents widen and open as the dyad blossoms into glorious smiles, or the sharp bodily aversions, painful cries, and the desperate expression of infants' bodies overwhelmed and going limp with fright when the interaction is cut off or disrupted. This co-experiencing arises from the "between," from the immersion of both the infant and caretaker in the compelling bond. Again, "These capacities to distinguish self, others, and objects refute the primary narcissism or egocentrism set forth by Freud and Piaget (1928) ... The neonate does not start from a self-centered state but is self-with-others from the very beginning" (Fuchs, 2013, p. 666).

The infant's awareness of self and others is actualized through keenly sensitive, multimodal sensory perception. As early as in the first months, relying heavily on proprioceptive awareness of their own body and the proprioceptive discernment of the other through posture, movement, facial expressions, and gestures, infants can discern emotion (Trevarthan, 2005). Additionally, the tactile distinction of self-touch and the touch of and preference for the touch of another (Rochat & Hespos, 1997), voice recognition of the other, and discernment of smell of the other all come into play in the infant's capacity to discern self and other as well as the emotional expressions of self and other.

An infant's awareness of interactions with another is present from the very beginning:

> Recent evidence for the presence of mirror neurons and adaptive oscillators along with the deepening literature on early imitation suggests that, probably from the beginning of life, infants have the capacity for what Braten (1998) terms altero-centric participation or what Trevarthan (1979) has long called primary intersubjectivity ... The implications for affective resonance, imitation, intersubjectivity, and empathy are evident.
>
> (Stern, 2018, pp. xix–xx)

Adaptive neural oscillators permit us to synch our movements to those of others and remain in synchrony with the timing of another's movement (Port, Cummins & McCauley, 1995). Such findings underline the long-perceived infant and adult's capacity to feel another's action and act accordingly in an age-appropriate fashion. Findings show that infants perceive perfect contingency and distinguish high but imperfect contingent relations, that is, precise matching rhythms of expression in, for example, vocal, bodily, and facial expression. The same findings show that by three months, however, they prefer high but imperfect contingency. This implies that generated movements by others become more interesting to the infant than perfect mirroring of their own movements. These neural responses are heightened in parent–child dyads revealing the neural underpinnings of attachment (Pratt, Goldstein & Feldman, 2018).

While infants experience first-person self-authority regarding primal experiences such as comfort or discomfort, hunger, and thirst, *the meaning of these feelings only comes alive in a shared context.* Winnicott (1989[1970]) articulated how affectively attuned interaction between the mother or caretaker and infant is required for an infant to attain embodiment. He described how this occurs as the mother or caretaker introduces the psyche to the soma through emotionally attuned articulation of the infant's feeling states being communicated to the baby over and over again. Though he was working from a developmental model in which the infant's task was to differentiate from the mother to establish autonomy as an individual, he nonetheless identified the essential interactions that led to what he described as psyche coming to dwell in the body (Winnicott, 1961). The later research of Stern and others on infant development fleshed out Winnicott's premise of how it is that happens. Most significantly, how *the meaning of the infant's innate capacity to feel only comes alive in a shared context.*

Sensorimotor experience organizes and is metabolized by the infant within the interaffective matrix of the infant–caretaker dyad, giving rise to another experience that can be formulated as meaningful affect. The infant internalizes these experiences as patterns of "ways of being with" as psyche comes to indwell the soma. Winnicott perceived self or ego development originating here—as an imaginative elaboration of body experience.

Stern's research underlines that these domains of self are not relinquished as further development unfolds; instead, they become substantive aspects of self that come in and out of the foreground throughout life.

In the psychotherapeutic process, the core sense of self can be accessed through *affectively attuned* exploration. I have found that when attuned responses incorporate bodily-felt sense access to the core, physical sense of self is heightened.

Affect attunement is distinct from empathy. While both kinds of response begin with emotional resonance, attuned responses communicate the nonverbal musicality, that is, the amplitude, rhythm, and at times the gestural expressions indicative of "*feeling along with*" another. Such moving along with and through is typically non-conscious or implicit. Rather than the traditional stance of analytic neutrality, the analyst conveys a sense of being with and moved by the analysand (Boston Change Process Study Group, *from this point forward* BCPSG, 2018). While such responsiveness may be subtle, it is a nonverbal, active acknowledgment of embodied interaffectivity. In contrast, though emotional resonance is foundational to both, empathic responses communicate *understanding* of emotion or meaning.

Winnicott described the interactive field between the analyst and analysand as a holding environment. This interactive field is cultivated between the analyst and the analysand as early states of mind are encountered and reworked. When bodily-felt sense and sensation are folded into affectively attuned response, I have found that it adds dimensionality, substantializing the presence of the body of the analysand. Most experienced, affectively oriented therapists offer attuned responses all the time without thinking much about them—it is a natural way of being with a patient's feelings. Attuned responses facilitate bringing coherence and soothing to the core sense of self, much as a mother or self-regulating other does with an infant through actual holding and attuned physical touch. When things go well enough, touch and physical holding is the predominant aspect of relating with infants and young children within the domain of a core sense of self. In the context of depth psychotherapy, touch and holding are beyond the limits of the "talking cure" interaction. Historically, in part because of this, the body has gone missing from the cure. The primacy of the body in psychic life and relationship requires that the bodily basis or the felt sense of intra- and interpsychic life be brought into *felt awareness* in the analytic unfolding. Frequently, this can be accomplished through the analyst's awareness of their own body and bodily-based relational experiences in the analytic engagement accompanied by simple expressions of sustained attunement to the core sense of self.

These dyadic interactions allow the patient to cultivate a capacity to attune to self, engendering the inner security of secure attachment. Through such interactive processes, the analysand also develops more capacity to attune and respond to another. Over time, this capacity for embodied self and other reflection reworks disturbances in attachment patterns (Siegel, 2020). In this manner, the analyst's quality and mode of affective response, including affective congruence in the words spoken to repair dyadic disruption, are psychophysically internalized by the analysand, and new (intra- and interpsychic) working models are formed. This illustrates the BCPSG formulation that "Psychoanalytic treatment can be viewed as the catalyzing of new capacities as patient and analyst move through the patient's most troubling vulnerabilities in increasingly fluent and flexible ways, as communicated most immediately through body-based interaffectivity" (BCPSG, 2018).

3.   The Sense of a Subjective Self

Between the seventh and ninth months, infants gradually recognize that inner subjective experiences—the intention to act, the desire to be held, or fascination with a toy or butterfly, all the subject matter of their "mind"—are potentially shareable with someone else. This brings about the recognition that she has an inner subjective world or "mind," and that other people do as well. At this early phase of development, the subject matter is minimal, such as an intention to act ("I want to touch the cat!"). Alternatively, communication of a feeling state ("This is so exciting!") or a shared focus of attention ("Look at it jump!") is what the infant senses is understood by another. This amounts to the acquisition of what is referred to as a "theory" of separate minds. When infants sense that others, distinct from themselves, can hold a subjective state, such as a feeling, thought, attention, or intention, that is similar to theirs, intersubjectivity is possible. (Stern refers to this as secondary intersubjectivity. It is distinct from the primary intersubjective nature of relating present at the beginning of life.) Of course, this is not a full-blown theory in the adult sense of the word. Stern, having a great feel for infants, refers to it as a working notion that goes something like this: "what is going on in my mind may be similar enough to what is going on in your mind that we can somehow communicate this (without words) and thereby experience inner subjectivity" (Stern, 2018, p. 124).

That this communication is unfolding nonverbally underlines that its occurrence is only possible because of the sense of meaning shared through gesture, posture, intonation, and facial expression. Interpersonal interaction begins to move from overt actions to internal states behind overt actions. Sensing this shift, parents and others begin to relate to the infant from this more subjective domain, adding more verbal responses to the subjectivity embedded in the nonverbal cues of the infant. With this leap, a new organizing subjective perspective about the self emerges.

It is truly remarkable how the emergence of a more autonomous self coincides with a newfound capacity to relate with an other. Emphasizing that this intersubjective relatedness is built on the foundation of core relatedness, Stern says:

> Core relatedness, with its establishment of *the physical and sensory distinctions* of self and other, is the necessary precondition, since the possibility of sharing subjective experience has no meaning unless it is a transaction that

occurs against *the surety of a physically distinct and separate* self and other. While intersubjective relatedness transforms the interpersonal world, however *core-relatedness continues. Inner subjective relatedness does not displace it; nothing ever will. It is the existential bedrock of interpersonal relations. When the domain of intersubjective relatedness is added, core-relatedness and inter-subjective relatedness coexist and interact. Each domain affects the experience of the other.*

(Stern, 2018, p. 125, italics added)

This development heralds a very significant shift in the infant's interpersonal world. Now, empathic responses from the caregiver are not just registered by the infant but are felt to bridge inner experiences between the two. Empathy, which is so essential for the infant's development, now becomes a direct subject of the infant's experience. Psychic intimacy, with its openness to disclosure and permeability, can unfold. Psychic and physical intimacy are now possible. The desire to know and be known is powerful and can be felt as a need state.

Alternately, when interactive dynamics are troubled, an infant can nonverbally express a refusal to be known and, through this, experience a sense of power in the turbulent relationship. The expression of refusal is a fully embodied response. Beebe (2014) describes a pattern of refusal that, when apparent early in a baby's life, is a predictor of insecure attachment pattern, resistant type, at 12 months:

To every maternal overture, the infant could move his body back, duck his head down, turn his head away, or pull his hand out of mother's grasp, exercising a virtual veto power over the mother's efforts to engage him in a face-to-face encounter … Moreover, rather than tuning out, the infant remained exquisitely sensitive to the mother's every movement, an acute vigilance.

(Beebe, 2014, p. 9)

As the subjective self of the infant emerges, the socialization of the infant's subjective experience becomes an issue, whether conscious or unconscious; parental attitudes hold great sway here, as do cultural shapings. What part of the private subjective experience is shareable and what is not to be shared; how much is to be shared and what the consequences are of sharing or not—all come into play. The significance of this is no less than a sense of belonging at one end of the spectrum and cosmic isolation at the other.

Because these dynamics will play out over the years, some interactive dynamics will be explicitly remembered, but much will be laid down implicitly. This poses potent challenges to the analytic couple; not only is the psychic material that needs addressing unconscious, it is often not accessible through imagistic-based memory. Instead, it is imprinted in the body (Van der Kolk, 2014; Ogden et al., 2006; Fuchs, 2018; Schore, 2009). While many depth psychotherapists have a sense of how these realms can be accessed via enactments (Bromberg, 2011), the ability to engage with nonverbal body-based realms can be especially useful here.

Case Vignette: Rick

Bodies, our own and others, are an aspect of every moment of our lives. Not unlike the earth or the air we breathe, our bodies are so ever-present that we often overlook them. Our bodies become obstructed from our awareness by the emotions, thoughts, and internal states we find ourselves in, such that we are rarely aware of the process by which these states emerge. This absence was amplified for me in a dream that I had about a man named Rick, who came to talk with me about possibly working together after his relapse into substance abuse. Rick, a first-generation Asian American man, initially presents as affable and engaged. These qualities shape an identity that belies an underlying disconnection from self and others. He let me know about the unintegrated quality of these disconnected aspects relatively early in our work, when, with considerable shame, he revealed that at times he cross-dresses when he is alone. He had no idea how to integrate this part of himself, for which his wife denigrated him. The pressure she exerted on him led him to come to therapy. I was left troubled by our first meeting and, that night, dreamt:

> Rick is in a room. He is alone.
>
> He is about to engage in an experiment that, in the dream, I know pertains to the theory of mind.
>
> Before him, on a flat, raised surface, there are five cups.
>
> His task is to choose the cup under which there is an eagle.
>
> He lifts each of the five cups.
>
> He comes up empty.
>
> There is no eagle.

I awoke numb with a kind of despair. It took me some time being with the image and the experience that hung in my body to begin to sense and formulate the feeling engendered in me by the dream, which was that of a vacuous emptiness.

In the dream, there is no body—no-bodied person present. Because there is no other, as would be necessary for the theory of mind experiment, Rick has no information on which to base a mental prediction of another's perspective, which is the experiment's premise. No-*body* there whom he could *sense* in a moment of shared attention. No-*body* there from whom he could glean an intent, much less a shared intent. In the dream, he proceeds to guess, or maybe he simply explores all options. He lifts each cup. He finds no eagle. No *body* of an eagle.

In the dream, I fully anticipated that the eagle would be found. That Rick comes up empty—that not only is there no other person but also no eagle to be found under any of the five cups—was, for me, while dreaming the dream, the last straw. Amplifying the feeling of emptiness in such a powerful way that I was left stunned, unable to think or feel. The disturbing dream and the bleakness it engendered lingered.

The dream helped me formulate my affect in Rick's presence. It also brought up the emptiness I feel in a world we are creating in which animal life, including eagles, is drastically diminishing. Eagles abound on video screens, but there are now fewer eagles to encounter body to body in our waking world. I am keenly aware that thoughts and fantasies about an eagle can never reproduce the feeling I have had on encountering an actual eagle, and the sense that the eagle also had an experience encountering me. The primal sense of awe reverberated so deeply in every cell of my body that I am sure I will never forget it.

I associate eagle with a potency felt by its palpable sense of intent. To me, the dream seemed to suggest that, in Rick's life, he has had no-*body* with whom he could sense shared attention about some realm of his psychic life. An absence of the possibility of intersubjective sharing. When with me, he vacated his body.

Part of Rick's dilemma in waking life is that despite considerable education, he can find no work or direction that engages him. As a result, he repeatedly loses himself by attempting to support others in what they desire. Unclear about what he feels or thinks, other than a desire to use substances, he uses. When cross-dressing, rather than the familiar blankness, he feels aroused.

The dream gives an imagistic portrayal of the psychophysical dynamics of our first meeting that registered in me via mirror neurons and other associated mechanisms. At first it seemed to be informing me about the unconscious feeling state of my patient. Yet I was also aware that it had touched something I inwardly knew. At a bodily level, I sensed movement even though the dream image was a still scene. From Daniel Stern's perspective, the dream captured a form of vitality imprinted in both me and Rick—an emptying out, a void, a waning of a feeling of being alive. As I sat with it, more insight emerged. I linked this feeling state to one that I am revisited by and left struggling with every nine or ten years. The light went off inside when I linked it to the fact that I was nine years old when my father died. Stern refers to kinesthetically contoured emotions that lie just beyond our familiar lexicon of emotions as forms of vitality (2010). This emotion fell on the far end of the spectrum as it was markedly de-vitalizing.

A potent vein of the unconscious communication occurring between Rick and me was transmitted via bodily resonance evoking a blank empty feeling, a wordless shock. Working with the dream and the concomitant bodily-felt elements opened a portal, a *way in*, to bridge to that which Rick knew but could neither think or feel, what Donnel Stern (1997) refers to as unformulated affect and Bollas (1987) as the unthought known.

My emphasis here is on the feeling engendered *in me* via the dream and how it augmented my reflections on the embodied interaffectivity constellating our interaction. The classic interpretation of the theory of mind experiment is rooted in the Cartesian dualism in which an antagonistic gap exists between first-person and third-person perspectives, that is, between the observer and the subject. The observer infers the other's perspective based on the best hypothesis of the reasons and motives of the other's behavior; alternately, the observer comes to know the other's mind (perspective) via simulating within an as-if mental state of the other, as a way to figure out the other's perspective (a first-person process). While this antagonism between subject and object is embedded in the legacy of psychoanalysis, the relational turn aims to undo this approach. Heightening awareness of the bodily basis of the relational matrix furthers this aim.

In this way, an intersubjective perspective is derived from non-verbal, inter-bodily communication and resonant perceptions. From this perspective, "it is through our own bodily resonance and reactions that we become aware of the other in a particular way ... Through interactive coupling our body becomes the very medium of social cognition" (Fuchs, 2013, p. 5).

Following the dream, Rick revealed that he did not know how to deal with his emotions, so his strategy was to try to ignore them. The act of my listening to him kindled fear in him. Inwardly he was overwhelmed by a sense of not knowing what to do. When I asked what that was like for him in his body, he replied with fright that he felt numb all over. Sensing chaotic confusion (my thoughts began to tumble and whirl) embedded in the numbing, I gently encouraged him to let his awareness be with the numbness, suggesting that he could perhaps be with the felt sensations of numbness. While this was scary and unfamiliar, we were able to slow down the process enough that he could stay with and feel the numbness. By bringing his awareness here and sensing my interest, numbness dissolved into tingling sensations. With great vulnerability, he then expressed that he felt he could trust doing so with me. While this was very foreign to him, he also cherished feeling safe enough to do so. At some later point, he let me know that though he had never quite realized it, what he wished for most in his life was for someone to ask him what he was interested in. No one ever had. The whole process I regard as "moving through and being moved by" (BCPSG, 2018).

Notably, research has shown that those with an insecure attachment pattern do not perform as well on the false belief test (an aspect of the theory of mind experiment). Research has also shown that *sensorial perception* narrows for those for whom basic trust (an essential feature of secure attachment) has been disrupted (Fuchs, 2012).[2] This creates a negative feedback loop in which one over-speculates based on projection, fears, and traumatic beliefs because one cannot access the sensorial experience to allow one to assess others and discern if an other is trustable. In this vignette, Rick was able to reclaim his sensorial experience, which brought him into a direct experience of himself and his ability to sense my intent.

Secondary Intersubjectivity: The Sense of a Verbal Self

With language comes a new organizing self-perspective. In the second year of life, the emergence of language accentuates the creative act of self-discovery, opening a new realm of potential learning and interactive knowing. Now the young child can refer to herself as an objective entity. With this comes a capacity to reflect on oneself and shape a self-narrative. Children begin to imagine and represent things in their minds. Symbolic play emerges. The possibilities of knowing oneself and another through the joint sharing of attention, play, and learning exponentiate. Joint meanings are shaped and shared in a way not possible before. With the ability to imagine self as an object that can be experienced by another, and that can discern the (now objectifiable) other's inner state, comes the capacity for empathy.

Language acquisition and, along with it, symbolic capacity heralds a complexity in the realm of relatedness in which all of life's issues will be played out. The advance is monumental. However, it also poses a problem of integration for those aspects of self-experience and self-with-other experiences that are the implicit nonverbal elements of experience. Language does not eclipse core and intersubjective relatedness, but it can split it. A division lingers between what is able to be verbalized and shared and what remains experienced yet non-verbalized.

The predominance of amodal, bodily-based sensorial perception now becomes secondary. Yet, it remains a key element of implicit functioning in relationships and perceptions of others, particularly with the primary caregivers. For example, a child hears a choppy vocal cadence that she recognizes as her Mom. The single sensorial element constellates within, as it did when she was only months old, as a multifaceted recognition of her mother. This is amodal perception. Now, as a two-year-old, there are plenty of experiences and memories of her mom to draw on, but the choppy vocal cadence becomes the foreground element that sparks her perception. With the slight turning in of her shoulders, her ribs tighten, constricting her breath. Her hips and legs grip, matching the curling in of her shoulders and arms as she braces in anticipation of being related to in an unpredictable and choppy manner. Not wanting to upset the caretaker and make matters worse, she reflexively attempts to smooth out any discontinuity in the mood between them. Her eyes brighten, and she excitedly responds with words to the caretaker's suggestion that they have ice cream.

The child's bodily constrictions would most likely be imperceptible to anyone not trained in observational skills that track such subtle bodily expressions. This short vignette portrays a split unfolding between the verbal and nonverbal self. The nonverbal bodily self tightens and withdraws. The verbal self responds brightly with words that indicate a desire to join with the caretaker. Furthermore, as an adult, when scheduled analytic meetings are disrupted, she experiences this as being held in a choppy manner. This makes it hard for her to stay with her core sense of self— she loses continuity of awareness of her own well-being or its disruption, as well as an awareness of her emotional life.

The use of language brings its own perils as regards embodiment.

It also makes some part of our experience less sharable with ourselves and with others. It drives a wedge between two simultaneous forms of interpersonal experience: as it is lived and as it is verbally represented. Experience in the domain of emergent, core and inner subjective relatedness, which continue irrespective of language, can be embraced only very partially in the domain of verbal relatedness. And to the extent that events in the domain of verbal relatedness are held to be *what really happened*, experiences in these other domains suffer an alienation. (They can become the nether domains of experience.) Language, then, causes a split in the experience of the self. It also moves relatedness onto the impersonal abstract level intrinsic to language and away from the personal immediate level intrinsic to the other domains of relatedness.

(Stern, 2018, p. 304, italics added)

Words can be spoken, then reworked and respoken, deepening, furthering, and elaborating on experience. In this way, language does not recapture what has just occurred but furthers it, carrying experience forward, elaborating affect, meaning, and aesthetic appreciation. A deeper understanding becomes possible. Relational sharing allows one to unfold meanings that might not have been conscious otherwise. Cultural shapings can become more explicit (apparent). This is language at its ideal, but all too frequently, this is different from what unfolds. Words function to signify and categorize. The speed of language and our pace of life rarely allow the nuances of the actual lived moment to be brought into words. Even in the psychotherapeutic encounter, where the intent is to make room and give time for lived experience to be unpacked, much is lost in the service of understanding and the quest for meaning.

The multimodal sensorial realm inhabited by infants, poets, and many artists can be overridden in a single word. For example, an eight-year-old boy is outside playing in the garden while waiting for his friend. It is a warm spring day. He finds six roly-poly bugs. His friend arrives. Shoulder to shoulder, they kneel in the dirt and soon discover an extremely colorful caterpillar in the grass. Their eyes beam excitedly at each other. Together they make a box full of dirt and leaves for their caterpillar. When they come inside, the eight-year-old's father, who doesn't much like the neighbor boy, says in a cold voice: "Playing?" The warmth in his son's body seems to drain out of him immediately. His enthusiasm now diminished, they move on to building Legos, the friend now awkward and less fluid in the collaborative play.

The foundational nuances of the boys' relating unfold in a domain of experience not captured by the father's word "playing." Hurts that do not get repaired because they lie in the nether lands of experience, in the domain of the emergent, core, or intersubjective self, suffer isolation. Even the best attempts at repair can result in a confusion of misunderstandings.

As language develops, so does the familiarity of referring to oneself in both the first person and the third person. This gives rise to what might initially feel like an innocent knowing that one can be objectified, that is, represented in some manner different than one's subjectively felt sense of self. This development becomes apparent when a child begins to recognize that it is *he* that he sees in a mirror. Many developmentalists have marked this significant phase of a child's life because a new perspective of self blossoms. In our time, the widespread use of electronic devices brings this reality to a new height. Even very young children are familiar with their own faces represented on the screen, whether in a video conversation with another or in the photos or videos others take of them. Three-year-old children seem pretty adept at posing for a photo. It is not difficult to imagine the potential entrapments which may arise from this, including but not limited to acceptance and/or comparison of self to others and the potential of outwardly or inwardly generated (persecutory or glorifying) dialogue rooted in such objectification.

I will refer to this newly objectifiable self that comes with the emergence of language as the "conceptual self" in distinction to the "experiential self." While there are far-reaching psychological implications of the "conceptual self,"[3] the thrust of the therapeutic focus of this book concerns the "experiential self."

Case Vignette: Lucinda

Lucinda began analysis with me ten years ago in her early thirties. She was born in London, where her father's family had lived for many generations. Following the path of her father's line, Lucinda was highly educated. Her paternal grandfather had been headmaster at a strict and punitive all-boys boarding school. Her father was schooled there. The students bullied him. Signs of weakness shown to his father were met with vindictive physical discipline. Her mother's family is of Spanish descent, a heritage ravaged by decades of political turmoil, religious constraints, and sexual violence. When Lucinda was born, the mother had been in London for less than a year and felt desperately lonely for family and friends. Lucinda was left for long periods at the home of a beleaguered nanny, who herself had a young child.

Lucinda seemed to survive these early years by outstanding academic achievement and social conformity. As a young adult eager to shape her life, she moved to the United States to attend college in California. After graduating with honors in marine biology, she readily found work. Lucinda excels at almost everything she turns her attention to, although at times self-effacing about her abilities. She faces challenges with determination, successfully navigating tough situations. Caring deeply about the environment, she participated in research that led to preserving several threatened species off the coast of central California. She works well with others as her natural warmth helps colleagues feel at ease. By the time we began working together, although she had achieved a great deal professionally, she found it isolating. When she came out to her parents as lesbian, their disapproval and rejection were devastating. She struggled with compulsive eating. Her intense spiritual yearnings could find no resolve. She worked for a few years with a counseling psychologist who helped her with her eating problem. During this time, she dated and eventually fell in love with a woman she later married. Yet, a feeling of intense inner pressure dogged her.

She found her way to me, and we began analysis. While the longing for connection is a common manifestation of the anxiety engendered in attachment wounds, Lucinda's reflexive need to avoid disconnection potently colored her days (Lyons-Ruth, 2006). Drawing from Stern's developmental perspective, the scarcity of warmth and the early and persistent parental abandonment reverberated to the depths of her sense-of-self-in-relationship. Dissociative mechanisms brilliantly protected her inmost spirit from the overwhelming pain of those early years. Many psychoanalytic thinkers have attempted to describe that part of the psyche, that inmost spirit. Kalsched (2013) has referred to it as the imperishable spirit, Jung as the Self, and Winnicott as the true self. Therapists know well that protections that work to preserve that deep kernel of self-hood come at a cost. The very mechanisms that had protected Lucinda also affected her ability to integrate the complex affects and nuances of the nonverbal realm with her verbal world. This lack of integration affected her ability to be at ease with herself and with her intimate others, especially when they encountered the inevitable bumps that come with closeness. I will describe some of our work with the bodily-felt basis of her experience that helped with that integration, allowing her deep desire for connection to mature into relationships with more emotional depth.

At the onset of her analysis, Lucinda's deeply rooted strategies to avoid feelings of abandonment went by almost unnoticed by her. As her work deepened, it became clear how difficult it was to contact the feelings in these vulnerable realms. She had a great desire to be with the plethora of feelings she experienced on an ongoing basis, but frequently the descriptions about the situations kept us from contacting the feelings themselves. When I attempted to elicit the bodily-felt experience of feelings, with the hope of getting closer to her direct experience through the felt sensations of emotions, she reflexively redirected our attention to a different experiential domain. Her highly intuitive nature quickly went to other associated feelings and dilemmas. While this often led to generative exploration, I noted the pattern and kept my sustained attention on the underlying affect.

She spoke explicitly of the deep value in which she held her inner world of feelings and her desire to be with them. Lucinda *is* highly sensitive emotionally. Perhaps in part because of her innate emotional sensibilities, she needed a particularly sensitive holding and protection. This kind of protection was not supplied through early parental holding; rather, her memories of this were the opposite. She couldn't remember being held and felt frightened of her mother, who more readily turned away from, rather than toward Lucinda. Instead of having internalized a capacity to hold her own sensitivities, autonomous, self-protective mechanisms were almost always on the ready to serve to keep her and others from getting too close to her tender feelings within. Without her consciously knowing it, the reflexive shift away from direct experience distanced us from the terrified little one within who remained un-held and untouched. And it was this very closeness that she most longed for. In contrast, she did welcome my empathic reflections. What was safer than me feeling along with her through affectively attuned responses was knowing I could understand her feelings and accompany her along the way. She needed me to be the calming, soothing other—a much-needed idealized self-object. However, when there were empathic breaks, our efforts to repair these could be fraught. When we attempted repairs, Lucinda was inclined to get overtaken by the concrete details of what had transpired, leaving us both somewhat confused and disoriented. Frequently, these efforts were prone to move us away from feelings rather than resolve the upset in our connection.

During this phase of her therapy, fights that ensued between her and her partner could go on for days, leaving them both exhausted. Patching things back together was based as much on surrendering to the desire to stay together as it was on the result of actual repair of emotional disruption between them—or us. Over time, I came to understand that getting anywhere near feelings of relational hurt activated catastrophic fears associated with being physically disciplined and then abandoned for having expressed a need.

Being Felt and Feeling

Stern's research shows primary intersubjectivity in the earliest moments of life, in the emergent and core sense of self. In the intersubjective matrix, affects, by being jointly attended, take shape and become known as feelings to the child. Difficult affect unshared across nonverbal and verbal domains remains unformulated, leaving the child distant from this part of herself (and thus from others) as if in a numbing cloud of lostness. This imprints in the actual tissues of the body. For Lucinda, this manifested deep in the viscera and in a tensional field residing in the skin and its underlayer of surface muscles, particularly around her eyes and chest. Without further metabolization, such tension remains like undigested food in the gastrointestinal tract; it cannot break down, move through, and be taken up as nourishment or discarded as waste. In other words, the feeling cannot be consciously known and accepted (tolerated). It is like an unlived shroud is cast over a child's little body, what Bollas (1987) called the unthought-known and that we now often refer to as implicit memory.

Once feelings are felt within a responsive relational matrix, movement—meaning the way emotion moves and behaves in the whole organism—versus stasis is possible, allowing the child to go on being *fully in their bodies where psychological life unfolds without the disruption of unfolding time.* This is how I understand Winnicott's concept of "going on being" or Stern's "self-continuity."

Psychological trauma occurs when a child is not accompanied in, with, and through their feelings, leaving them with more feelings than can be metabolized (Russell, 1999). This can leave a child like Lucinda feeling utter aloneness. These words can be all too familiar, barely scratching the surface of the embodied actuality of the archetypal affect (Kalsched, 2013) of numbing aloneness. To apprehend the embodied reality, we have to drop down from the thinking mind.

One day, Lucinda entered my office seized by a fear that her withdrawn partner was having an affair. Any attempt to explore this hypercharged fear was met with deflection. Later, in the middle of the night, *I* dropped into a place of feeling that seemed resonant with what was too terrible for us to get near in that session. I awoke remembering and feeling myself as a little girl, alone in bed at night, haunted by something unnamed—a scary presence lurking in the night's shadows. As that child, I was too scared to call out. I imagined no help would come if I did. I remembered, or more likely my body remembered, the terror, and my body-self completely seized up. What arose in my awareness were times I would play "dead" with my younger sister, a game that often scared her to tears.

The grip of terror is a freeze response, a neurological response activated by fear. Feigning death is a furthering of a pre-reflective neurological response activated by the instinctual assessment that survival is severely threatened.

It is easy as a therapist to all too quickly become accustomed to word usage such that we no longer feel the meaning the words convey. For instance, here, in the words "neurological response, freeze, shutting down," we can lose track that those nerves live in the little child's body, and they create a cascade of stress hormones, muscular activation, images, and fantasies. Of course, the child *does not think this is a neurological event* or that she has unresolved, dissociated feelings. The experience is coursing through her, body and soul, but cannot be consciously known.

These middle-of-the-night rememberings in my body and the dream-like state were mine, and not mine. It is what got activated in my psyche-soma while working with Lucinda through the potent conscious and unconscious communications between us, including the neurological function of mirror neurons, adaptive oscillators, kinesthetic empathy, and affective resonance (Stern, 2018). It is an example of embodied interaffectivity that can unfold in the analytic engagement when encountering unformulated feelings. Part of the analyst's work is to help metabolize previously unformulated experiences of those with whom we work. Through bodily resonance, implicit, unformulated affect can find a path to consciousness if the analyst is attuned to their somatic unconscious. This is especially so when the unformulated painful feelings have some resonance in the analyst, though the content need not be similar. My experience, which I knew was linked to the period of stunned silence that reverberated through my family following my father's death, though very different in content from Lucinda's experience, offered me a path of empathic inquiry. By working through what it was like for me, in these feelings that lingered in my body, I could inquire from a place of felt empathy about her feelings of utter aloneness. Both of us were being worked by our coming together. Interactions like this between patient and healer/doctor/therapist (depending on cultural and historical context) have been recognized throughout history, and psychoanalysts discuss it most frequently in terms of projective identification. In the *Psychology of the Transference*, Jung writes:

> The patient, by bringing an activated unconscious content to bear upon the doctor, constellates the corresponding unconscious material in him, owing to the inductive effect which always emanates from projection in greater or lesser degree … the unconscious infection brings with it the therapeutic possibility … of the illness being transferred to the doctor.
>
> (1946, pp. 176–177)

Elsewhere, he writes: "The meeting of two personalities is like the contact of two chemical substances: if there is any reaction, both are transformed" (1933, p. 49).

Neuroscience extends our understanding of the bodily basis of such dynamics, offering us a way to think about what many clinicians experience. Jung's use of metaphor gets at what is happening yet remains beyond our clinical formulations. His use of metaphor creates a bridge to the emergent phenomena unfolding in the implicit intersubjective level of felt experience (Gendlin, 1995).

In time, Lucinda let me know how frightened she was of her body. This was so even though throughout her life, she had loved to dance. She belonged to a modern dance troupe and looked to movement as her source of sanity and well-being. However, exploration of what it felt like *inside* her body was a kind of forbidden territory. In time she was able to tell me how frightened she was of turning her awareness toward her breath. To her, inhalation felt cold, and with this arose unbearable and unformulated feelings. We came to understand that for her, coldness was synonymous with the feeling of aloneness. Fuchs describes the research that has shown how,

> affective qualities of a situation trigger a specific bodily resonance ("affection") which in turn influences the emotional perception of the situation and implies a corresponding action readiness ("*e-motion*"). Embodied affectivity consists in the whole interactive cycle which is crucially mediated by the resonance of the feeling in the body ... Bodily felt warmth thus directly affected the interpersonal impression of warmth ... Interpersonal coldness was thus felt as physical coldness.
>
> (Fuchs, 2018, pp. 124–125)

Over time, Lucinda was able to bring attention to what her feeling states were like inside—and I learned to rarely use the words "body" and "sensation," or to inquire directly about her breath. I might often ask if there was an image of what it felt like inside. If something arose, I might ask about the felt sensation of the image. Alternatively, I might simply gesture to a place on my body while asking what's it like inside her.

At one point, not long after we had repaired, well enough, a disruption between us that had occurred, she had a very upsetting experience with her wife. As she recounted her experience, we slowed down the telling, and she found a way to tell me more about what it was like *inside*. She was able to tell me of the pain she experienced in her chest. She sensed the pain was linked to her anxious feelings, but it frightened her, making exploring them even harder. She feared there was a lurking problem with her heart. Staying with the sensations gave way to a more discernable sense of a tight pulsing dread. By being with ever so tiny amounts of the felt sensations, there came a gradual relief of some of the tension and fear.

Yet a sense of a low-lying terror persisted. Her fear became so urgent that it seemed evident to us that it did not belong to the current situation only (Davies, 2005). She suddenly recalled a recent dream:

> *I am in a dark forest. I have a wooden contraption that I put over this woman's head who is coming toward me. It rests down on her shoulders. It has a long protruding handle. I can hold the handle to keep her from getting too close. She is so scary. I let her near in one moment, and the woman sinks her long claw-like fingernails into my hand.*

She drew a parallel between her feelings toward the woman in the dream and those she felt toward her partner when she behaved in a withdrawn manner. Quickly following this, she remembered feeling really scared of her nanny and her mother when she was little. Her nanny, not unlike her mother, would turn away and not respond when Lucinda most wanted and needed connection. Based on stories her family shared, Lucinda knew that, especially in the first months of her life, her mother often left her with the nanny, sometimes for days on end. It was hard to access and remember her early feelings about her mother because, now, she and her mother had done a great deal of work to transform their relationship. Her current feelings seemed the antithesis of those feelings. But the experience of her spouse abruptly cutting her off, and the scary woman in the dream, revivified body-based memories from the past.

Making these links helped her to stay in relation with me. We were able to slow down the flood of feelings and be with them in micro bits, titrating the highly charged traumatic sensations and feelings such that she could feel moments of genuine emotion rather than be flooded and panicked by feelings that manifested as a flood of stories. In this way, she remembered the dissociated feelings belonging to the little girl who would awake frightened and run to her parents for comfort. She would be taken back to her room, spanked hard, ordered to stay, and left there in her room. She cried from a place deep in her core. The tears came from the young, terrified little girl within.

She then was able to tell me that this same inner pressure in her chest was what she had felt when we had been talking about the disruption that had occurred between us. This again brought more relief from the terror, somatically felt as pressure. Of equal importance was that something that had been un-sharable found a relational home between us.

Something shifted following these sessions. Less entangled in this traumatic complex, she was more able to inhabit the adult self within, such that she could reflect on and comfort this frightened child part when it arose again. Now I could inquire if her adult self could, in her imagination, be with that scared little girl. She readily shifted into this imaginal realm and held the little girl in her lap and against her chest. To further access the somatic dimension of her imaginative process, I gently inquired if she could (imaginatively) sense the weight of the little girl as she held her in her lap. We did not encounter any of the typical obstacles when, with a light-handed, slow-paced yet sustained attention to the fine details, I inquired about her somatic experience: "What do you notice in your body as you do this? How is the little girl sitting—facing front or nestled up against your chest? Do you sense the contact as pressure or warmth? Is it comfortable or uncomfortable to have her there? Can you say a little bit more about what you notice in your body that lets you know this?"

She settled more fully in her body as she responded to the inquiries that resonated with her. She was able not just to imagine but simultaneously be with the accompanying felt sensation of the imaginative process. Her adult self acknowledged, validated, and comforted the five-year-old little girl who had been frightened *out of her body* into uncontrollable catastrophic fantasies. The little girl could settle, no longer highjacked by the terror that had gripped her body in a dissociative freeze state while she simultaneously fled (Levine, 2010) through the runaway (verbalized) fantasies of a terrified five-year-old now packaged in an adult's world. This time around, the story had been about her wife leaving her, cascading into fears that her niece, who was having a hard time, would also break off connection with her and she would be all alone in her old age. We had become familiar with stories (from the verbal self) cascading like this and came to refer to them as *feelings looking for a story* (feelings of the nonverbal self).

In this manner of working together, as empathic repairs were imperfectly but continually navigated and trust was built between us, something began to shift. An example of this came when, during an analytic hour, an inner imperative would arise, as if from Lucinda's depths. With a soft but urgent certainty, Lucinda would suddenly announce that she needed to pause and feel her body. She came to articulate that this was necessary to avoid running over herself with her own words. We would both enter into moments of silence during which she would turn her attention inward to bodily-felt sensations. At first, it felt important that I let her inwardly explore on her own while remaining silent yet attentive. This began to occur more frequently during our time together. Though at first we did not talk about the specifics of what happened in her inner exploration, she would return to her narrative and engage in a different pace, one that left more room to be with her inner experience and feelings as opposed to reporting on the urgent details of her life. She would recognize when she needed to slow down her speaking to feel, and she could initiate this. From this place, her feelings seemed more palpable to me, and I could, in turn, respond with more substance and depth of reflection. As this happened, her intrapersonal exploration deepened, accompanied by increased insight and the maturation of her relational capacities with me, her partner, and her friends. She began to crave working from this deeper dimension.

Once, when she was lying down, she all of a sudden reported to me that she felt her whole body in an important connection to the earth. I asked her with the simple words "*if it is okay*, just notice the weight of your body." After a pause, I added "as if you were lying on a beach and your body made an indent in the sand." As she let that happen, she reported a deep settling in her chest, as if there had been a swirling wind there, and now it was quieting, and the back of her chest settling, allowing space to open in the front. She told me this was like floating in the warm ocean on a moonlit night. She spoke of experiencing a bubble rising into her chest, and with that came a big breath and a feeling of reassurance about her niece. She told me she could feel a deep peace opening inside her.

We explored how her fear that something catastrophic would happen to her niece was rooted in intergenerational trauma. A hallmark of being caught in the vortex of intergenerational trauma is the inability to have a perspective on the future. This perspective let her settle within even more deeply, allowing us to continue to be with the feelings that were beginning to find a place to be felt and integrated within rather than projected onto the next generation, as was done to her and her two brothers.

I am still moved by the quiet miracle of that moment when she turned within and connected to the earth, her body, and the tender parts of herself and me. Something synergistic that was greater than both of us emerged. This is what Ogden (1994) referred to as the analytic third. Jung (1977/1970) called it the *coniunctio*—the union of the opposites: between her rational mind and her body, between her and me, and between her and the greater earth. With that union came the birth of new possibilities: an unfolding in her heart shifting the earlier awful pressure to a felt sweetness through a radical acceptance of feeling.

Later, in other sessions, she told me about different scenarios that engender the horrible feeling inside of being a bad person. We explored how this pressure drives her to do everything possible to disprove that feeling. Nevertheless, it constantly haunts her. We continued exploring the corrosive effect on her as a little girl of being constantly judged and punished for being perceived as bad. We explored it as the best formulation her young self could make to ensure she maintained a connection to her mom—as long as she could imagine she could do better, be "good," she had some control and hope in preserving that connection. We explored how that was arising between us in her proactive approach to discussing what she was struggling with and how, at times, this approach often distanced us from her more vulnerable feelings. I reflected on the fine line between meeting her where she was and colluding with this autonomous defensive function. For example, I might enter a session conscious of this dynamic between us, yet once immersed in her concerns, I found it hard to navigate our interaction differently without potentially shaming her in an attempt to bring her awareness to what might be happening between us. Our interaction put a flame under my awareness of our situation.

A few weeks later, she was lying on the couch in such a way that if she opened her eyes, we could make eye contact. She had entered the room highly agitated and was trying to calm herself down. She tells me she is so scared. At this moment, I feel more like I am in the presence of a scared animal than an adult or a little girl. I let her know this. We talk together about how animals have feelings too. I asked her: If an animal had been treated like she had been, trapped, hit, and told it was bad, over and over again, how would she be moved to be with it? She says she would just be present, give it space, food, and water, hoping it would start to trust her a bit. Then she blurts out, "It is all physical!" I ask her what it is inside that she is noticing. She reports tightness in her face, eyes, heart, and shoulders. With our attention focused on felt experience, we enter the immediacy of the moment, sharing in the heightened, careful quiet she has described she needs. She tells me that there is a feeling of space opening in the interior cavity of her heart area. I can see she is quieting, and I feel the shared resonance of a sense of space to be in, to inhabit. With a softening voice, she again tells me how frightened she has been of the pain and tension in her chest. Then she tells me that the animal needs time—with no expectation that it needs to get better or change. Just to be.

She draws a circle in the air above her face and chest—tracing it in both directions—clockwise and counterclockwise. In time she says it is a sacred circle. I ask her what color. A gold orb, she responds. I ask where she feels herself to be in relation to it. "Inside it," she replies. I ask, what happens inside you when you feel yourself within it? In time, she says, "I can let down." I say something like, "sorta like all the cells inside can start to settle?" She says, "Yeah, I get this is the part of me that is often gripped and tremulous when I am here with you." I ask her if she is feeling safe here with me now. She says, "Today, yes, now, enough. But I do not think being this slow (inside) when I am out and about in the city is possible."

In later sessions, we returned to the glow she felt from the gold orb—an archetypal image and experience of wholeness—rather than fragmentation and disconnection—an ancient place of healing. Doing so helped her sustain the felt interiority and a link to hope for the future. As new neural networks had been laid down, the felt image and our shared attention to it served as an ongoing invitation for her psyche to reside here, to indwell, to be in this state of wholeness. I think of this as the ongoing process of mending the traumatic disruption of her core self with her verbal self (Stern, 2018). This is what Winnicott (1970) described as occurring when the caretaker introduces the child's psyche to her soma, over and over again, allowing the child's psyche to come to indwell the soma.

As the psychophysically based emotional working through settled, and she was no longer in a fragmented state, she reflected on her highly developed verbal capacity. She recounted how she determinedly got into a college in the United States and earned a Ph.D. She described how she sought to excel academically, as a dancer, and in all other ways possible in order to be above reproach. She spoke of how pursuing an education had been so important to her. It situated her "above reproach" and afforded her a healthy path out of the dark, confusing emotional chaos she had grown up with. While we had come to recognize that her use of words had been reflexive, a protective mechanism aimed at distancing her from feelings that were too overwhelming to deal with on her own, it also deserved appreciation because it had truly saved her (Kalsched, 2023). Her siblings had not fared as well, having been caught up in extreme promiscuity that had led to bad marriages and domestic violence, or malignant identification with victimization. She recognized it took her a long time to avoid overriding her feelings with words. However, she realized that working with traumatic memories from these depths affected a far-reaching transformation relative to exploration of the same material through talking alone (verbal sense of self).

As we spoke of this, more insights arose about her earlier dream. Though terrified in the dream, she also found a way to protect herself. She recognizes how she uses words to keep others, including me, at a distance, particularly if she feels she is criticized or is not being seen. The dream helped her own the fact that she does to others the very thing she feels they do to her—keep them at a distance. Reconnecting with these projected shadow elements proved to be empowering. She felt less prone to feeling overtaken by an urgent need to be "right" when hurt was activated. This let her slow down and soften in relation to others, including me.

Our work exemplifies the dimensionality of felt experience that could not be accessed with words alone. The overuse of words sabotaged attempts to deal with the traumatic activation and truncated what she most desired—to be connected and understood.

Reflecting on Stern's Clinical Applications

Clinically applying his research findings, Stern encourages us to be attentive to the domain of self-experience most prevalent in a patient's narrative. He has seen how discerning which sense of self (emergent, core, subjective, intersubjective, or verbal) is suffering could be the most salient clue to the narrative point of entry of an individual's inner world, enhancing and quickening the therapeutic process. For instance, recognizing Lucinda's difficulty being with her core sense of self, and inviting her to be with the felt sensations of her own weight, helped her shift from a verbally dominated narrative and land in her actual felt physicality. This is important because by settling into her felt sense, she becomes present in the here and now, experiencing and reflecting on her subjective experience rather than talking about herself as an object. Furthermore, it allowed us to work directly with titrating the highly charged traumatic activation. In these moments, transformation is possible (BCPSG, 1998).

If her concerns had been about self-agency, and she had described being ordered to "not move," or if she had experienced being "physically restrained," then inquiries directed towards the physical experience of "moving" or "restraint" could likely have been good entryways into her implicit memories. Domains of experience come in and out of focus throughout life, as well as within one analytic hour; thus, the emphasis is on linking with the most prevalent domain rather than a specific developmental phase or stage (Stern, 1985). Initially, what mattered most to Lucinda was knowing and feeling I was with her, ameliorating the terror of abandoned aloneness. Thus, empathic inquires and responses helped forge a bond with her intersubjective sense of self.

Braiding the Nonverbal and Verbal Worlds

Stern describes how the emergence of a verbal sense of self enables one to articulate various aspects of experience and thus come to know oneself and be known in a fuller way than ever before. Knowing and being known becomes utterly compelling because we are innately oriented to connect. The urge to discover and dialogue about the wider world can be insistent and fascinating. So, too, is the discovery of and sharing of one's inner mythopoetic world. Lucinda began to discover this realm as lived in her body. Something emerges when both the nonverbal and verbal self are found and woven together. A young Navajo man once told me that his grandfather taught him that their people's braided hair represents the interweaving of body, emotions, and spirit—how strong and beautiful they became when braided together.

Reawakening to the Nonverbal World

Stern's research dramatically enhances our understanding of the nonverbal world and underlines how the nonverbal realm does not disappear as an individual matures into adulthood. Infants make sense of their world and learn about their caretakers through sensorial abilities that are nothing short of remarkable. Language gathers thoughts, reflections, and emotions into a temporally organized mode of expression. Our task as psychotherapists is to maintain integrity in our use of language. It is possible to bring forth the sensorial realm rather than categorizing and displacing it as belonging only to children, poets, and artists. Without reflective integrity, language can be overly linear, organizing not just thoughts and feelings into a linear template but bodily movement as well. Because many of us think and learn in nonlinear kinesthetic, auditory, or imagistic ways, this can give rise to shame when it does not match the dominant mode of organizing expression. Chapter 2 addressed how other cultures place much more emphasis on sensorial knowing.

The acquisition of language and the range of what is permissible to talk about varies immensely in individuals, families, and cultures. In an earlier clinical vignette, Rick said, "I do not understand or know how to talk about my emotions, so I ignore them." In so doing, nearly the entire emotional domain was off limits to Rick, significantly narrowing his subjective sense of self.

While one's cultural and familial attitudes shape what gets attended to, there is much the body knows, at a less than conscious level, about direct experience. Sensorial perception shapes how one experiences and acts within the environment and with those in our surroundings. Much of this knowledge remains implicit, shaping affective response, the concomitant sensorimotor impulses, and how we inhabit our bodies.

The nonverbal world is atmospheric and ever-present, and because of this, it may be easier to grok its significance by entertaining its absence. Imagine a redwood forest that remains utterly silent, with no shifting currents of wind whooshing through its branches. Imagine a dog that does not bark and whose body, face, and tail remain motionless. Imagine lightning with no thunder. Imagine a soundless evening despite an abundance of cicadas nestled in cottonwood trees. Imagine an infant rigidly and robotically discovering their first words. Recall how hard it is to witness the recent experiments in which we see and feel the utter distress an infant experiences when his mother or father goes still-face (Tronick 2007, www.youtube.com/watch?v=YTTSXc6sARg). Imagine a world where holding an infant is delegated to Artificial Intelligence: www.instagram.com/reel/CnpzghBBlRK/?utm_source=ig_web_copy_l

Working with the body in depth psychotherapy invites one to reinhabit the vast, fascinating, and somewhat mysterious nonverbal world.

A Guided Practice to Bodily-based Experience

Here is a guided practice to explore the gap between the verbal and nonverbal domains of experience. If you feel drawn, you might see what you find when you have a quiet moment.

What more does your body want you to know about this?

The next time you feel yourself a bit out of sorts emotionally, consciously inhibit the impulse to analyze, figure out, fix, or find its historical roots.

Turn your attention inward; you might let your gaze soften or close your eyes to do this.

Notice what's happening in your breath. Perhaps it's jagged, faint, or restricted.

Allow your attention to be with your breath without trying to change it; just be with it as it is.

In a short time, with your attention, your breath will inevitably begin to adjust. Just let that happen.

Notice how it does so without direction from you but happens simply by virtue of your attention.

Now, notice the felt experience in your chest area, your arms, and your hands.

Now, notice your lower abdomen, pelvis, legs, and feet.

Notice the sensations in your head, perhaps within the cranium itself, as well as your face, eyes, jaw, and mouth.

Do you feel constriction or tightness? Laxity or collapse? Or maybe a heaviness or churning?

Notice the texture and quality of your inner experience.

Does it feel jumpy, racing, staticky, stagnant, or perhaps edgy?

Ask your body—these qualities you are experiencing—such as the heaviness or edginess itself, if they had a voice what they want to tell you. What do the qualities want you to know?

Imagine these qualities as a person you are interested in getting to know.

Try to give your body the time it needs to find its own words.

Stay with your breath as if it were a flashlight, illuminating this lesser-known part of your experience.

Notes

1 While similar such pathological entities do exist later in life, these findings clarify that they do not have their origins in the first two years of life, uprooting the clinical notion that regression to these states is a pathogenic mechanism.

2 While autistic children may derive a third-person perspective by repetitive learning of others' regularities, this lacks the second-person perspective of knowing the other through interactive bodily affective resonance, where our emotions unfold and gain meaning.

3 See Feher et al. (1990) for in-depth and expansive foundational perspective.

References

Beebe, B. (2014). My journey in infant research and psychoanalysis: Microanalysis, a social microscope, *Psychoanalytic Psychology, 31*(1), 4 –25.

Beebe, B., Cohen, P., & Lachmann, F. M. (2016). *The mother–infant interaction picture book: Origins of attachment.* D. Yothers (Illustrator). New York: W. W. Norton.

Beebe, B. & Lachmann, F. M. (1988). The contribution of mother–infant mutual influence to the origins of self and object representations. *Psychoanalytic Psychology, 5*(4), 304–337. https://doi.org/10.1037/0736-9735.5.4.305

Bollas, C. (1987). *The shadow of the object: Psychoanalysis of the unthought known.* New York: Columbia University Press.

Boston Change Process Study Group (BCPSG). (1998). The process of therapeutic change involving implicit knowledge: Some implications of developmental observations for adult psychotherapy. *Infant Mental Health Journal,* 19(3), 300–308.

———— (2018). Moving through and being moved by: Embodiment in development and in the therapeutic relationship, *Contemporary Psychoanalysis, 54*(2), 299–321. https://doi.org/10.1080/00107530.2018.1456841

Braten, S. (1998). Infant learning by altero-centric, participation: The reverse of egocentric, observation, and autism. In S. Braden (Ed.), *Intersubjective, communication and emotion in early ontogeny.* Cambridge: Cambridge University Press.

Bromberg, P. M. (2011). *The shadow of the tsunami and the growth of the relational mind.* New York, London: Routledge.

Davies, J. M. (2005). Transformations of desire and despair reflections on the termination process from a relational perspective, *Psychoanalytic Dialogues, 15*(6), 779–805. https://doi.org/10.2513/s10481885pd1506_1

Driscoll, R. (2020) *The sensing body in the visual arts: Making and experiencing sculpture.* London, New York: Bloomsbury Visual Arts.

Feher, M., Naddaff, R., Crary, J., Foster, H. & Tazi, N. (Eds.) (1990). *Fragments for a history of the human body* (Three volume set). New York: Zone/MIT Press.

Fuchs, T. (2013). The phenomenology and development of social perspectives. *Phenomenology and the Cognitive Sciences, 12*(4), 655–683.

———— (2018). *Ecology of the brain.* Oxford: Oxford University Press.

Gendlin, E. T. (1995). Crossing and dipping: Some terms for approaching the interface between natural understanding and logical formulation. *Mind Mach, 5*(4), 547–560. https://doi.org/10.1007/BF00974985

Jung, C. G. (1933). *Modern man in search of a soul.* New York: Harcourt, Brace.

———— (1946). *The psychology of the transference. Collected Works, Vol. 16.* Princeton, NJ: Princeton University Press.

———— (1977/1970). *Mysterium coniunctionis. Collected Works, Vol. 14.* Princeton, NJ: Princeton University Press.

Kalsched, D. (2013). *Trauma and the soul: A psycho-spiritual approach to human development and its interruption.* New York: Routledge.

Levine, P. A. (2010). In an unspoken voice: How the body releases trauma and restores goodness. Berkeley: North Atlantic Books.

Lyons-Ruth, K. (2006). The Interface Between Attachment and Intersubjectivity: Perspective from the Longitudinal Study of Disorganized Attachment, *Psychoanalytic Inquiry, 26*(4), 595.

Mahler, M. S., & Furer, M. (1968). *On human symbiosis and the vicissitudes of individua-tion*. New York: International University Press.

Ogden, P., Minton, K., & Pain, C. (2006). *Trauma and the body: A sensorimotor approach to psychotherapy*. New York: W. W. Norton.

Ogden, T. H. (1994). The analytic third: Working with intersubjective clinical facts, *The International Journal of Psychoanalysis*, *75*(1), 3–19.

Port, R. F., Cummins, F., & McAuley, J. D. (1995). Naive time, temporal patterns and human audition. In R. F. Port & T. van Gelder (Eds.), *Mind as motion: Explorations in the dynamics of cognition* (pp. 339–372). Cambridge, MA: MIT Press.

Pratt, M., Goldstein, A., & Feldman, R. (2018). Child brain exhibits a multi-rhythmic response to attachment cues, *Social Cognitive and Affective Neuroscience*, *13*(9), 957–966. https://doi.org/10.1093/scan/nsy062

Rochat, P., & Hespos, S. J. (1997). Differential rooting response by neonates: Evidence for an early sense of self. *Early Development and Parenting*, *6* (3–4), 105–112.

Russell, P. (1999). Trauma and the cognitive function of affects. In J. G. Teicholz & D. Kriegman (Eds.), *Trauma, repetition, and affect regulation: The work of Paul Russell*. London: Rebus Press.

Sander, L. W., Nahum, J. P., Harrison, A. M., Lyons-Ruth, K., Morgan, A. C., Bruschweiler-Stern, N., & Tronick, E. Z. (1998). Non-interpretive mechanisms in psychoanalytic therapy: The something more than interpretation. *International Journal of Psychoanalysis*, *79*, 908–921.

Schore, A. N. (2009). Right-brain affect regulation an essential mechanism of development, trauma, dissociation, and psychotherapy. In D. Fosha, D. J. Siegel, & M. F. Solomon (Eds.), *The healing power of emotion: Affective neuroscience, development & clinical practice*. New York: W. W. Norton.

Siegel, D. J. (2020). The developing mind: How relationships and the brain interact to shape who we are. New York: Guilford Press. 3rd ed. (Kindle Edition).

Stern, D. B. (1997). *Unformulated experience: From dissociation to imagination in psychoanalysis*. El Dorado Hills, CA: Analytic Press.

Stern, D. N. (1998). The process of therapeutic change involving implicit knowledge: Some implications of developmental observations for adult psychotherapy. *Infant Mental Health Journal*, *19*(3), 300–308.

———— (2010). *Forms of vitality: Exploring dynamic experience in psychology, the arts, psychotherapy, and development*. Oxford/New York: Oxford University Press.

———— (2018/1985). *The interpersonal world of the infant: View from psychoanalysis and developmental psychology*. New York: Basic Books.

Trevarthen, C. (1979). Communication and cooperation in early infancy: A description of primary intersubjectivity. In M. Bullowa (Ed.), *Before speech: The beginning of interper-sonal communication*. New York: Cambridge University Press.

———— (2005). Action and emotion in development of cultural intelligence: Why infants have feelings like ours. In B. D. Homer & C. S. Tamis-LeMonda (Eds.), *The development of social cognition and communication* (pp. 38–58). Mahwah, NJ: Lawrence Erlbaum.

Tronick, E. (2007). Still face experiment. www.youtube.com/watch?v=YTTSXc6sARg.

van der Kolk, B. (2014). *The body keeps the score: Brain, mind, and body in the healing of trauma*. New York: Viking Press.

Werner, H. (1948). *The comparative psychology of mental development*. New York: International University Press.

Winnicott, D. W. (1961). The theory of the parent–infant relationship. *International Journal of Psychoanalysis*, 41, 585–595.

———— (1989/1970) On the basis for self in body. In C. Winnicott, R. Shepherd, & M. Davis (Eds.), *Psychoanalytic explorations.* Cambridge, MA: Harvard University Press, pp. 261–283.

Zahavi, D. (1999). *Self-awareness and alterity. A phenomenological investigation.* Evanston, IL: Northwestern University Press.

Chapter 5

Forms of Vitality

Alexis is a trans person—female to gender nonbinary—who likes to be called "Alie" or "Alex," and to be referred to by the pronoun "they."

When we began working together, Alie was employed in a nonprofit organization that focused on immigrant rights and social services. The organization introduced Alie to a form of inner work focused on embodied activism and leadership. The foundation of this approach to personal growth and leadership was to align with one's own embodied self and move into the world from a place of grounded, personal clarity. Useful group practices helped them gain a way of understanding their own self-protective strategies in a bodily-based way. Alie felt these tools gave them a way to navigate the sometimes bumpy ride of their interior life. Alie was aware of their tendency to be judgmental of themselves and others, and how this sometimes triggered contempt. There had been times when Alie would fall into depressive episodes that nearly incapacitated them. Because the self-help tools and group work they had learned in this professional training were so useful, they were left disoriented when the depressive episodes hit and the tools were not enough to shift their mood.

Alie's father was a Christian missionary, which required the family to move every four to five years when Alie was young. Alie grew up in Guatemala, Nicaragua, and Micronesia, and felt they had been well cared for and provided for as a child. Education was prioritized, and Alie did well academically. While there was much Alie appreciated about having tasted the richness of other cultures, Alie had become aware of how others' beliefs often conflicted with the beliefs and demands they had been taught in their family and religious community. The overarching conflict was rooted in the degradation of bodily life, especially toward women and sexuality. Because of the danger believed to stem from women's sexuality, children being held or touched after the age of two was not condoned. Their mother was judged as indulgent if she physically comforted or held Alie or their sister.

The family returned to the United States for Alie to attend college in California. Once Alie graduated, they made a life for themself in the San Francisco Bay Area. Within a few years, based on what had begun to arise regarding Alie's sense of self while in college, they transitioned, identifying as gender nonbinary. Alie

DOI: 10.4324/9781003305804-6

found companionship and a long-sought sense of community within the LGBT community.

When Alie began dating a Nicaraguan woman with whom they worked, Alie felt passion arise in a way they had never known. They spent a few tumultuous years together. Alie was no stranger to separation, so when their girlfriend abruptly decided to return to Nicaragua, Alie forged ahead despite the pain and confusion.

A year later, Alie fell in love with another woman, and they married. Alie felt that their life as a couple was good. Their wife had often complained of wanting more physical and sensual contact. Alie was aware that their wife's pleas had a triggering effect on them, but it felt murky and confusing. Rather than being able to emotionally process with their wife, some part withdrew even more from physical intimacy. However, Alie felt their daily companionship, shared social values, and engaged community life far overrode the sense of something missing. When their wife revealed she was in a sexual relationship with another person, and that that person was a man, Alie was devastated and came to work with me.

A pivotal experience occurred a few years into our work. Alie had been struggling to untangle difficult feelings about their self. Now, a mood of depression hangs over them. During this time, I experience Alie's vitality to be like a pond in what would usually be a lush landscape that is now rain-starved. Scattered plants on the hillside that would be green this time of year now appear an odd grey. Here and there, branches jut down toward the water with brown and crinkled leaves in a way that is disturbing in its unexpectedness. Seeing the colors this way, my heart cringes, and my eyes search for the continuity of meadow life I expect to see in this verdant landscape of the person I know as Alie. It is like I can smell the too-still air at the pond's edge and feel the agitation in me caused by the bugs hovering on the pond's stagnant edge. There is a constriction of flow, the vitality that my eyes anticipate does not come through Alie. The constriction of flow between us has become palpable. I see Alie searching with their eyes, almost leaning forward and pulling back simultaneously. Searching, yet alone and very still inside. I feel a vertical grip extending from my chest down beyond my solar plexus. Alie tells me how, for hours each night, they lay awake and scroll through their social media, but it only worsens the emptiness.

As we sit in the silence, I wonder aloud if they might scan their body. I say: "By scan, I mean turn your attention inward and let your awareness drop in and sense each inner region from the top down. As you get a felt sense of yourself from the inside out, notice if something arises that gets your attention."

I see Alie's hands shift, clench, then open slowly. I softly suggest that they stay with what they notice happening in their hands and listen to what wants to happen. I see Alie attending to something inside; I suggest that no matter how subtle, just listen. In time, I add, listen for what wants to happen, stay with it, and listen for what more your body knows about this.

Alie's hands rise to their face as if to cover their eyes. As Alie's hands find their eyes, I see their hands soften and drift down the skin of their face, and for a long moment, they touch the skin of their cheeks very tenderly. A tear wells in the corner of their left eye. Their hands slowly move down their face to their heart and linger there. Now their hands come down to their thighs, and a tear falls. Almost imperceptibly, their hand strokes their thigh and then rests in their lap.

Alie looks up from this very internal place and finds my eyes. When Alie speaks, their voice seems to emerge from another realm, distant yet immediate, saying, as they again touch their face, "These are my eyes ... this is my heart ... my sex, not no-body's or some-body else's."

I feel a quivering inside, so touched by Alie's vulnerability. I let them know this. We sit in this pregnant silence for a long, little while. Maybe I sigh in resonance occasionally, but no other words are spoken. No other words seem necessary. The session ends.

The next time we meet, Alie tells me that this experience lingered inside over the next few days, and at some point, a song emerged that they had heard long ago. Tentatively, Alie spoke a few lines of the song, *The First Time Ever I Saw Your Face*.[1] Their voice and body subtly vibrated with a feeling of awe, a genuine experience of intimacy—with themselves—as they expressed the tenderness evoked by the song and their embodied memory of touching their own face, heart and sex.. For Alie, this intimacy was an encounter with the true self, dwelling within their own felt body. Alie told me that, for the first time, they actually *felt* their body alive and to be their own. Alie said, "*I feel real.*"

I watched the release of the subtle but unmistakable flow that had been constricted; their vulnerability emerged. The tender place they entered also inhabited the shared space between us. Though shy, Alie was making contact with me. I could feel a new dimensionality to Alie's presence, a sense of them being behind their eyes.

Grieving followed for what had been lost and forbidden between them and their mother, and their father as well.

The pond source no longer constricted, Alie's vitality emerged, with the kind of seasonal rhythms recognizable in the going-on being of personhood. It was in the matrix of our relationship and my being with them, witnessing them, that they could make contact with a direct experience of their self, their body.

Later through our dialogue, Alie understood that the contrast between what others conceived Alie's body to be, or what Ali conceived or even wished their body to be, was very different from this experience of actually feeling, from the inside, their own body. In touching their own body, Alie felt touched. A portal opened. Alie began to feel an acceptance of their bodily self that seemed completely new, what Winnicott referred to as an experience of true self (1960).

Movement Is Life

This experience initiated Alie's reinhabiting their body, yet it was not a static body. Alie contacted the movement that is inherent to life. I saw the color return to their face. I felt the energy flow through my own body as the opening occurred for Alie. I heard it in the words of the song.

Movement may be as subtle as the cellular vibrations of tonicity. I could see this had diminished in Alie, and this had been jarring as it sharply contrasted the liveliness I had come to know in them. Within any specific movement is a force. Vitality is the force manifested in all living things. In death, as was so with the brittle branches and their brown shriveled leaves, nothing moves.

Our ability to read or imagine another's thoughts, emotions, and "will" depends on motion. Before this event, I could sense I was "losing" Alie. They seemed very far away. After weeks of constriction, the return of their vibratory aliveness was like the return of spring for me, and for Alie.

Understanding Forms of Vitality

Inherent to the notion of an embodied mind is that all acts must take on a temporal shape. Without this, the human world is nonrecognizable, not incarnated (Stern, 2010). Intensity, direction (intention), duration, and spatial contour, are the forces that course and shift through our bodies and are intrinsic to all movement, what Stern refers to as the "form of vitality." Before the "why" and "what" of an event is the "how," from a body-based rather than conceptual perspective. Our organisms register the dynamic of action, such as gentle, holding still, surging, pulsing, or retreating. These are not emotions.

> They are not sensations in the strict sense, as they have no modality. They are not direct cognition in any usual sense. They are not acts, as they have no goal state and no specific means. They fall between all the cracks … They do not belong to any particular content … They concern the "How," the manner, and the style, not the "What" or "Why."
>
> (Stern, 2010, p. 8)

"They are psychological, subjective phenomena that emerge from the encounter with (the) dynamic events" (2010, p. 7) of emotion, thought, and sensation. They are primarily expressed by adjectives and adverbs, and give emotions, sensation, and thought a sense of their quality, direction, and force. They can also convey the quality of a particular person at any given time. Contemporary neuroscience inquiries regarding the source of this activation in our bodies are ongoing, and tend to focus on the arousal system (Stern, 2010).[23]

Body-based Inquiry and the Movement of Vitality

This is why it is not enough to ask someone where they feel something in their body. When we take the inquiry further, asking someone to stay with the felt awareness in their body by noticing what it is like and what happens next, we are contacting the quality, contour, and movement. In this way, we can contact the form of vitality intrinsic to the moment, even in states subjectively perceived as strangled, as with Alie. Daniel Stern emphasizes that, "affect attunement is based on matching and sharing, dynamic forms of vitality, but across different modalities" (2010, p. 42).

Most therapists pursue this kind of inquiry in an affectively attuned manner, though we are not usually conscious of just how it is that we are doing so. Recognizing that one's attunement may be expressed in the timing of one's facial expression, as well as verbal intonation, can bring an added dimension to how we think and reflect on what it is we are doing.

Pursuing this kind of inquiry in an emotionally attuned manner constitutes a microanalysis of moment-to-moment direct experience, what the Boston Change Process Study Group (Bruschweiler-Stern et al., 2018) refers to as the local level. Sustained attention to the immediacy of experience reveals more of the feel of its inherent vitality, whether a tightening (in force and direction), stasis (a description of time), or sense of color or image (shape).

These aspects of expression offer a *way in* to what otherwise may seem elusive and uncontactable, what Donnel Stern (2018) refers to as unformulated experience. It is this lived dynamic that is more than affect, more than thought or reflection, that the BCPSG illuminates as intrinsic qualities of implicit relational knowing. Exploring this realm "may be useful in reorienting some of our notions of emotion theory, memory structure, social communication, as well as psychotherapeutic theory and practice" (Stern, 2010, p. 17).

A form of vitality underlies episodic memories and shapes the narratives we create about our lives (Stern, 1985; Lyons-Ruth, 1999; Bruschweiler-Stern et al., 2002). As we track the rise and flow of emotion within the person of the therapist or the analysand, or between the two, deeper insight can frequently be gained through the dynamics of the vitality rather than the content. For instance, what is it like to feel this deadness? Or this surging forth and falling back into sour constriction? Is it familiar? If so, when has it been experienced? What is your earliest memory of this pattern of feeling? "Forms of vitality are part of all past experience. As such, they offer a special verbal way to evoke past experience" (Stern, 2010, p.11). Verbal formulations arise, in part, from specific inner sensorial experience and the felt sense of the gestalt of inwardly felt experience (Gendlin, 1969).[4][5] This kind of inquiry might lead more directly into the affectively charged patterns of being with another, non-conscious experience, implicitly known and never verbalized.

As Alie and I continued to explore their experience in these ways, painful moments in their early life emerged. As a young child, Alie longed to be comforted and held by their mother. Although Alie had some notion that their father, and the Christian community they were part of, forbade such physical touch, deep down, Alie had come to believe that something was wrong with their body. Over time, Alie's body often felt far away. As a teen, in sexual explorations, Ali had very disturbing episodes of somehow not feeling real, which clinically we refer to as depersonalization, a form of dissociation.

Affects Imprint in the Body in Time and Continue over Time

Dynamic contours of affect live in the body in a moment in time, and over time. Though joyful feelings may linger, they do not seem to lodge in the body–mind, whereas difficult feelings often do. They require more of us, and more effort to stay with when we do not like them or are instinctually motivated to move away. Conscious reflection is required to work through or "move along" through such feelings. If left "unfinished" or "unresolved," they linger and imprint in our bodies, even as we (consciously) forget. This is particularly so of affects engendered in pervasive developmental trauma.

Feelings that a child cannot metabolize can leave them in a mild but pervasive state of dissociation. Consciously, what remains is the gnawing feeling that something is not quite right within. For example, when Alie's mother would not hold them despite Alie's need, powerful feelings would surge through Alie—such as anger, rage, hate, sadness, and despair. Alie needed their mother, needed to be held. In the face of this shattered expectation, Alie needed somehow to preserve a sense of an attachment to their mother. Rather than hating their mom, which would have left them feeling desperately alone, Alie's hateful feelings turned inward; Alie blamed themself. Something must be wrong with them. Otherwise, their mother would hold them. Over time, Alie found themself hating their body. Their sense of body image was confusing and negative. Alie's ability to speak their thoughts was, at times, also hampered, and this, too, was confusing. These outer manifestations of their inner pain were glaring, but the inner pain, now dissociated, had become unidentifiable. Shame overtook their bodily based sense of self.

From a Jungian perspective, dissociated affects such as these accrue archetypal valances, manifesting in images, dreams, and symptoms. This kind of inner psychic territory is familiar territory for depth psychotherapists. What I want to emphasize here is the way *affects, shaped by their particular form of vitality, go on living in the body. Affects are more like movement phrases than a single moment's event.*

The form of vitality that shapes the "how" of an affect is not described in the primary affects articulated by Darwin. They come through in words like exploding, swelling, rushing, relaxing, languorous, effortful, gentle, fading, tentative, tightly. Common enough words, but they are neither pure emotion, strictly sensation, nor pure perception. The Latin root of emotion is *emovere*, to move out. Here we get a feel for how the force of vitality within an emotion registers within—though sometimes out of awareness—as an impulse or as an initiatory muscular readying that, within a micro-moment, is allowed or inhibited. Expressed perhaps as a fisted hand pounding a table in anger, a child skipping with joy, the sunken cheeks and dropped jaw of loss, the almost imperceptible muscular grip about the spine when registering disagreement, a sadness stirring about the heart, or the spontaneous desire to hug a loved one following a long separation. The shape, contour, and tempo of vitality affects are a dynamic in motion that continues to live within, imprinting in posture and subtle and not-so-subtle movement patterns.

Like a musical phrase, the vitality form of an affect plays out in the body. Unfurling the bodily-based afterlife of an emotional phrase can help bring one out of the isolating capsule of trauma. The unfurling frequently carries meaning forward, reframing the original trauma as one discovers how it gives rise to meaning, creativity, and purpose (Bollas, 1995).

Archetypally, this may be variously expressed as the phoenix rising from the ashes of psychic death, or in the transformation of the chrysalis to butterfly, or as Demeter rising from the underworld renewing life's growthful energies. These storied images express a dynamic continuum. When brought to consciousness, such a continuum can literally be felt in a painful unfolding of tissues in the body and in the awakening of a pulsing awe. Awe has a vital form—one is moved.

The Default Mode Network and Cultivating Vitality after Trauma

Staying with this unfurling shape, tempo, and contour of affect as it unfolds in the body and takes on the mythic dimension of meaning is essential in processing trauma.

We know that the processing of developmental trauma lays down new neural networks, allowing new behavioral and relational possibilities. Yet in clinical practice, even after a great deal of interpersonal and intrapsychic work has been done, it is not unusual to hear those who have experienced severe, pervasive developmental trauma finding themselves caught up in a tangle of memories or feelings that lead to a swamp of devitalization or the swirl of overactivation. These states are often particularly pronounced upon waking. Neuroscientific research has identified that the Default Mode Network (DMN) is a network of brain regions that are active when our minds are at rest, and we are not focused on a specific task. It activates when an individual engages in introspective activities such as daydreaming, contemplating the past or the future, or thinking about the perspective of someone else. Default Mode Network is known to be atypically active in those who have suffered trauma. Pervasive developmental trauma can bias the DMN towards re-experiencing traumatic events, associated feelings, and beliefs (Hajong, 2021).

Cultivating a gateway back to a felt sense of possibility can help the individual navigate those discouraging waters of the DMN, though at times more processing of specific traumatic memories may be in order. Contemplative mindfulness practices such as focusing on breath and body sensations have been shown to mitigate the overactivation of DMN and bring one's focus into present-centered awareness. Mindfulness engages two circuits in the brain. One is a lateralized experiencing circuit associated with knowing through direct experience. The other circuit involves awareness of, or the conscious witnessing of, what we know (Farb et al., 2007). Continued practice facilitates "distinguishing the many forms of the 'known' such as enhancing the ability to stably perceive feelings, thoughts, and memories with curiosity, openness, acceptance, and positive regard" (Siegel & Gottman, 2015, p. 216).

Alie's Song

The internalization of an inner witness emerges from having been sufficiently witnessed by a compassionate other—often this is the therapist. Using our relationship as a basis, Alie was able to turn inward and see–feel their body in a new way.

Once Alie internalized and further developed their capacity to witness themself, they were able, when alone, to turn inward on purpose, in a kind and nonjudgmental way. Alie found singing the lyrics of the song, accompanied by the gentle touch of their hand to their cheek, to be a *way in* and through these kinds of difficult states when they re-emerged (Bollas, 1992). Their attuned self-witnessing furthered the cultivation of *earned* secure attachment within (Siegel, 2007).[6]

Simple yet profound acts such as tenderly touching one's own cheek or bringing a contemplative attitude to a wide range of body-based practices such as walking, yoga, meditation, or everyday tasks can shift the organism's inner organization out of the residues of the traumatic vortex that lingers in the default network toward vitality.

The Jungian process of Active Imagination is a paradigmatic approach. Neuroscience research has revealed that when we imagine movement, the same regions of the brain associated with actual movement and emotions are activated, leading to new neural connections. When a word is heard, such as "skip," signals register not only in the language centers of the brain but also in sensorimotor regions and areas involved in the actual enactment of the word.

> When someone imagines a movement with its vitality form, something happens in the cortex that then sends a signal to the appropriate motor areas to activate the musculature of the body that would've been used if the imagined event were enacted.
>
> (Stern, 2010, p.133)

The imagined movement comes alive in the flesh of the body. Furthermore, mental models and neural networks can be reshaped by doing something differently, imagining it differently, feeling it differently, seeing another's way of doing it or hearing about it in words. Alie soon found it equally transformative to sing silently within and imagine their cheek touched. What is paramount in shifting implicit relational knowing is the direct act of doing, sensing, feeling, or imagining differently rather than talking about it.

Notes

1 For the lyrics, written by Ewan MacColl (1957) and sung by Roberta Flack, go to: https://open.spotify.com/track/0SxFyA4FqmEQqZVuAlg8lf.

2 In addition to the arousal system, Stern explores the possible neurological systems involved in vitality forms, including the sensory-motor system. He describes a wide spectrum of the ways forms of vitality are involved in movement, imaging, language, and intersubjective experiencing, all of which illuminate the embodied basis of apprehending the other as occurs in the therapeutic dyad (Stern, 2010, pp. 45–55).

3 See the Zone Books, in particular, *Zone 3: Fragments for a History of the Human Body, Part 1, The Expressiveness of the Body and the Divergence of Greek and Chinese Medicine*, which explores the profoundly different ways of understanding and experiencing the phenomenon of vitality between two cultures (Kuriyam, 2000).

4 Eugene Gendlin's (1969) "*Focusing*" is an eloquent approach to eliciting verbal expression sourced from the gestalt of the felt sense of experience.

5 Stern (2010, p. 49) describes how Gallese and Lakoff (2005) extend our understanding of the entwinement of the sensory-motor system and language formation by explaining how, "through a process of 'neural exploitation' sensory motor mechanisms have, during evolution, taken on new roles in imagining, concept construction, and language. This upsets the traditional view that concepts and language are abstract, symbolic, amodal and arbitrary and are assembled in another 'third place' (e.g., a language center) ... These functions, too, are assembled in the sensorimotor system, and in this way become 'embodied'."

6 The neurological system engages when we bring *attention* to intention. When one is attuning to the intentional state of another person, such as a parent to a child or therapist to patient, a state of *interpersonal* attunement is created. When one brings attention to one's own intention, such as following one's breath in meditation, a state of *intrapersonal* attunement is created. These states engender the deep sensations of fullness and stability that occur with resonant and harmonious states of mind. These states of interpersonal and intrapersonal attunement promote internal security and coherence in one's sense of self, as is characteristic of secure attachment. See Siegel and Gottman (2015, pp. 173–174).

References

Bollas, C. (1992). *Being a character: Psychoanalysis and self experience*. New York: Hill & Wang.

———— (1995). *Cracking up: The work of unconscious experience*. New York: Hill & Wang.

Bruschweiler-Stern, N., Harrison, A. M., Lyons-Ruth, K., Morgan, A. C., Nahum, J. P., Sander, L. W., Stern, D. N., & Tronick, E. Z. (2002). Explicating the implicit: The local level and the microprocess of change in the analytic situation. *International Journal of Psychoanalysis*, *83*(5), 1051–1062.

Bruschweiler-Stern, N., Lyons-Ruth, K., Morgan, A. C., Nahum, J. P., & Reis, B. (2018). Moving through and being moved by: Embodiment in development and in the therapeutic relationship. *Contemporary Psychoanalysis*, *54*(2), 299–321. https://doi.org/10.1080/00107530.2018.1456841

Farb, N. A. S., Segal, Z. V., Mayberg, H., Bean, J., McKeon, D., Fatima, Z. & Anderson, A. K. (2007). Attending to the present: Mindfulness meditation reveals distinct neural modes of self-reference. *Social Cognitive and Affective Neuroscience*, *2*(4), 313–322.

Flack, R. (1972). The first time ever I saw your face. Written by Ewan MacColl (1957). Source: LyricFind.com.

Gallese, V., & Lakoff, G. (2005). The brain's concepts: The role of the sensory-motor system in conceptual knowledge. *Cognitive Neuropsychology*, *21*, 1–25.

Gendlin, E. T. (1969). Focusing. *Psychotherapy: Theory, Research & Practice*, *6*(1), 4–15.

Hajong, D. (2021). *The role of the default mode network in post-traumatic stress disorder*. Delhi: University of Dehli, Lady Shri Ram College for Women.

Kuriyam, S. (2000). *The expressiveness of the body and the divergence of Greek and Chinese medicine*. New York: Zone Books.

Lyons-Ruth, K. (1999). The two-person unconscious: Intersubjective dialogue, enactive relational representation, and the emergence of new forms relational organization. *Psychoanalytic Inquiry*, *19*(4), 576–617. https://doi.org/10.1080/07351699909534267

Siegel, D. J. (2007). *The Mindful Brain: Reflection and Attunement in the Cultivation of Well-Being*. New York: W. W. Norton.

Seigel, D. J., & Gottman, M. (2015). An interpersonal neurobiology approach to developmental trauma: The possible role of mindful awareness and treatment. In V. M. Follette, J. Briere, D. Rozelle, J. W. Hopper, & D. I. Rome (Eds.), *Mindfulness oriented interventions for trauma: integrating contemplative practices*. New York, London: The Guilford Press.

Stern, D. B. (2018). *The infinity of the unsaid: Unformulated experience, language, and the nonverbal*. New York, London: Routledge.

Stern, D. N. (1985). *The interpersonal world of the infant: A view from psychoanalysis and developmental psychology*. London: Routledge

——— (2010). *Forms of vitality: Exploring dynamic experience in psychology, the arts, psychotherapy, and development*. Oxford: Oxford University Press. https://doi.org/10.1093/med:psych/9780199586066.001.0001

Winnicott, D. W. (1960). Ego distortion in terms of true and false self. In D. W. Winnicott (Ed.), *The maturational processes and the facilitating environment: Studies in the theory of emotional development* (pp. 140–152). London: Karnac Books.

Chapter 6

Languaging the Body

The body is ever present, pulsing, sparkling, seething, receding, disappearing, reaching towards gripping, freezing, melting, effervescing, whether one is alone or with another, whether thinking, perceiving, or feeling. "The living body is the very possibility of contact, not just with others but with oneself—the very possibility of reflection, of thought, of knowledge" (Abrams, 1996, pp. 45–46). How do we bring integrity to our language so we do not further the polarization of body and mind? Poets and children often do this seamlessly. Naomi Shihab Nye, in her poem, *One Boy Told Me* (1998), gives voice to the embodied musicality a boy wants others to know he experiences when he bursts forth, telling us that music lives inside his legs and that's what comes out when he talks! The boy's experience can help us apprehend what Gallese's and Lakoff's (2005) research reveals of the entwinement of the sensory-motor system and language formation. They explain how "through a process of 'neural exploitation' sensory motor mechanisms have, during evolution, taken on new roles in imagining, concept construction, and language. This upsets the traditional view that concepts and language are abstract, symbolic, amodal and arbitrary and are assembled in another 'third place' (e.g., a language center) ... These functions, too, are assembled in the sensorimotor system, and in this way become 'embodied'." (Stern, 2010, p. 49).

We, psychotherapists, cannot change the polarizing tendencies embedded in our culture's use of language or undo centuries of the subtle and not-so-subtle effect of valuing the mind as though it had no body and no need for a body. Still, we can strive to re-infuse our language, as does the boy in the poem, with the subjective nuance of embodied life that has been concealed at the same time as the objectification of the body and subjugation of bodily-based experience have been imposed.

The body speaks persuasively without words. We understand its language though we may only rarely be aware of all it is we "hear." At times, in analytic practice, my inquiry and responses may be directed to the felt experience of the body. Yet the body is always present, whether addressing felt sensation or the verbal expression of intra- and intersubjective experience. How can my language reflect this? Historically, the language of psychoanalysis often amplifies the split between body and mind. The words "mind," and even "psyche," often connote the part of the person that is separate from the body. Specific concepts such as mentalizing further accentuate polarization.

DOI: 10.4324/9781003305804-7

In addition to languaging the body, can we learn to track the moment-to-moment unfolding at the implicit or bodily-based level to enhance our relational acuity and make our work more efficient (Bruschweiler-Stern et al., 2002)?

Our wordless sensorial experience is in constant play with imagination and reverie, and this interaction makes way for creative ways of knowing and perceiving. Even when referring to the body as a metaphor, it is the real heart that is inextricably bound to the neurological basis of emotion that goes on beating and feeling whether one is aware of feeling or not.

As we have seen, emotions are neurologically based and felt through the sensorimotor system. Emotions belong not only to the individual but are shared states felt through bodily-based interaffectivity (Fuchs, 2018). The BCPSG refers to interaffectivity via the phrase "moving through and being moved by" (Bruschweiler-Stern et al., 2018). These words have a musicality that evokes inner kinesthetic referencing. The BCPSG emphasizes how the meaning-making process itself arises as one moves through the world and is moved by another and, I would add, the world itself. In this way, meaning-making is a participatory unfolding. They articulate that:

> First, we move to an embodied language of therapeutic treatment because the body speaks eloquently through movement, intention, and affect.
>
> Second, we register the other body's language largely outside of consciousness and move through the orientation of another in terms of our own embodied resonances.
>
> Third, we enter the minds of others through this embodied moving-through process in which we participate in the other's intentions and attitudes.
>
> Fourth, we view the therapeutic process as one not merely of resolving conflicts but as one of catalyzing new capacities for relationship. In this regard, the embodied moving through process in psychotherapy drives the long developmental trajectory involved in coming to know our own and others' minds.
>
> Fifth, this moving through process also drives the development of new capacities for relationship when undertaken therapeutically in an engaged relationship with a positively charged other. We chose the term "moving through" from current thinking about embodied communication. … The process of moving through is grounded in action and also encompasses the process of being emotionally moved by the other in relational encounters.
>
> Interaffectvity, being seen, known, felt. This combination of action and feeling is critical to interbody communication.
>
> (Bruschweiler-Stern et al., 2018, p. 300)

By foregrounding the significance of the biological body in intersubjective relating, the BCPSG expands and deepens perspectives on psychoanalytic treatment written about by Freud, Jung, and many contemporary relational psychoanalysts. They emphasize how embodied resonances occur through mirror neurons, adaptive regulators, and other neurological dynamics. As we relate to others, *our* neurological systems register *their* micromovements and affects. In effect, at a nonconscious level, we are constantly experiencing the others' expressions, affects, and intentions in our own bodies. Fuchs and Koch (2014), whose perspective is not limited to the neurological but includes the sensorimotor system, in the tradition of Merleau-Ponty, refer to this as an intertwining that occurs in all our relationships. In ongoing relationships, there is a "trying on" of the other's attitudes toward self, and an implicit pull to integrate the other's take on the world into our own. The resultant inner friction can instigate a struggle to integrate or differentiate, which offers a potential reorganization of what was before.

The ongoing mirroring experience generated in us by the other at a nonconscious level that evokes in ourselves the other's intentional movements and affective states is the basis of attunement, which is distinct from, but inevitably contributes to, feelings of empathy. These interaffective processes are foundational to an embodied theory of mind. Empathy involves understanding the other's emotional situation as if it were one's own. Empathy has been far more studied than attunement. Attunement refers to feeling along with the other, resonating—perhaps it is more akin to dancing, and empathy more to verbal dialogue.

One could view the analytic encounter unfolding in two parallel dimensions—the verbal and the nonverbal. The verbal dimension comprises the usual components of psychoanalytic therapy, including what brings the analysand to seek therapy. It explores and clarifies this, understanding its roots, the issue in the context of the person's life, and as it lives between the analytic dyad. It examines what arises from the unconscious through dreams and imaginal processes, and listens for the prospective currents emerging. The other parallel dimension is the bodily-based and nonverbal. This unfolds in the bodies of both dyad members, their posture, facial expressions, gestures, and idiosyncratic modes of expression, and how these shift in innumerable and subtle ways as feelings arise and move along. The sense of momentum in the relational flow between them, such as a flooding of content by one or the other, or of emotion or its lack, the jaggedness, deadness, the ebb and flow of eros, the terse tension of what is unspoken, as well as bursts of laughter, are all aspects of this dimension.

A shared goal, though it may not be explicitly known, is a key element of the couple's intersubjective sharing. They may agree and differ on elements that comprise the goals. When disruption occurs via an empathic miss, lateness on the part of either, collision with their defenses, or collusion with a defense, these disruptions are the underlying intersubjective elements and feelings that require attention.

When the analyst is attuned to the nonverbal dimension as outlined above—not just intellectually but also in an emotionally authentic way—their body language, as well as their words, convey this. As a result, both the verbal and nonverbal dimensions have a chance of being contacted in the interaction.

Case Vignette: Róisín

My analysand, Róisín, enters and, unusually for her, remains silent, showing signs of perturbance. Her face is pallid, her mouth drawn, and her cheeks seem fallen and narrowed. She avoids direct eye contact. I remember Róisín had expressed outrage at the behavior of her wife, Elaine, in the prior session. At the time, I recognized by the level of her reactivity that a familiar feeling rooted in her traumatic past had been triggered. Rather than convey some empathy, I felt annoyed and impatient with the repetitive collapse of reflective awareness and concretization of Elaine's limitations. Sitting with my silent agitation, I aligned with her wife's point of view.

Now, as I sit with Róisín, I feel a kind of empty tightness in my chest. I notice, contain it, and say, "I am not sure, but you seem pretty tight and upset with me." She does not respond, and I say, "I have been thinking about our last session together all week. I wonder if my response about the clash you had with Elaine did not sit well?" If that had elicited a response like, "Yeah, I have felt really angry with you all week," we would have been back on track, with me conveying recognition that I "missed" her emotional upset at a time when she felt frayed and frightened by the ongoing difficulty they were having, amplifying her need for me to get it. From there, a dialogue might have opened in which we both explored our contributions to the interaction, and I expressed my regretful feelings about having missed the complexity of the exasperation, anger, and disappointment she had been feeling and how by doing so, she felt I had failed to grasp her.

However, that is not what happened. My attempt at exploring what had previously unfolded between us did not open the analytic space between us. Instead, Róisín shut down even more. Words seemed only to worsen the disconnect, as evidenced by the tense silence and stilted body language we were now both experiencing. After a short awkward silence, I tried to pivot. Aligning with her tempo and expression, I vocalized something like a soft grunt that, in a way, joined her, and asked if she could say a little bit about what it is like inside. She and I were familiar with this flavor of relational juncture between us. I could see she was processing her decision about what to do, and I saw her turn her attention inward. As she did, the rigidity in her body, characterized by her head jutting slightly forward and her fixed eyes demanding a response—a posture that conveys blame and injustice—softened. "I feel this squeezing in of my lower ribs. On the right more than the left. There is a pressure around my solar plexus … from not inhaling." I echo, "On the right … not inhaling." She blurts, "It is like that; I just want to get small … and not feel." She goes on to describe that, while growing up, almost any comment or behavior on her part would be met by her father's wrath. Grimacing in acknowledgment, I quietly encourage her to stay with the felt sensations a bit more and see what else she is aware of. She looks at me and then quickly away, saying she pretty much hated me all week. "Yeah," I respond, "when I sided with your wife, it felt pretty much like that, like I wiped out your feelings and point of view in one fell swoop, just as your father did." Nodding, Róisín's eyes water, her posture softens a bit more, and our dialogue opens.

In this way, bringing her awareness to the direct experience in her body offered her permission to be with the muddle that ensued from having to hold back her anger, hurt, and hate. The previous muddle of unformulated emotional experience found shape and contour. My willingness to receive the thrust of hate and survive (unlike her mother, who would disappear, or her father, who would retaliate with an annihilating force) opened a feeling of tenderness between us. Working directly with body-based sensation brings our attention to the unfolding moment, and now we are "moving along."

When Róisín first entered the room, I registered her body language and assessed my own inner state. I was not feeling empty and tight prior to her arrival. I wondered how much of what I was feeling resonated with what she might be feeling, or if it was my response to her inner state and the uneasiness it was causing in me. My own bodily-felt sense hovered in the background of my awareness as we spoke. Eventually, it led me to inquire about her bodily-based experience.

How Róisín shuts down in response to my empathic failure is a traumatic response imprinted in her implicit memory as a "way of being with an other," what the BCSPG calls implicit relational knowing (Bruschweiler-Stern et al., 2002). It is a pattern further held in place by a defense mechanism perpetuating the shutdown by insisting that either Róisín or I are to blame, and that it is best to say nothing rather than reveal her hurt and angry feelings (Kalsched, 2013).

From the perspective of "moving along," Róisín's affective state unfurled through our interaction. There were unpredictable moments of missing and refinding each other. However, we got through to a common-held goal of her gaining perspective on her past and the present. The outcome of this was an expanded relational capacity—as we loosened the entanglement, there was more room for her, myself, and her sense of Elaine as human and mucking about and making mistakes, as humans do. The grip of traumatically based implicit memories loosened, allowing a new experience and lessening the probability of her getting caught in this kind of traumatic vortex again (Levine, 2010).

The BCPSG states (with my additions in parenthesis and italics):

Although it has been a cornerstone of psychoanalytic theory that all behavior is motivated, it has never been considered at the level of intersubjective regulation in the domain of implicit knowledge at the local level [*the microanalysis of moment-to-moment activity occurring within each individual and between the dyad*]. We believe this level is an important addition and complement to traditional psychoanalytic concepts such as transference/countertransference and the unconscious ... Moreover, a great deal of the information that both analyst and patient gather about each other and their relationship derives from the implicit domain. Unless this is acknowledged, much of what transpires in an analysis will be missed.

(Bruschweiler-Stern et al., 2002, pp. 1059–1060)

An analytic process incorporating direct bodily-felt experience complements the dialogue of more familiar attuned responsiveness and interpretation, and is woven into it. The BCSPG refers to this as "the something more than interpretation that leads to change" (2002, p. 1052). These interactions facilitate the patient finding a greater perspective on life. Such an experience will always be accompanied by affect. When the analyst genuinely participates in the affect, "a moment of meeting" occurs (2002). Such an experience not only helps a patient regulate highly charged affect, as is often the aim of trauma interventions, but also sets in motion a new "way of being with another"—affect that seemed unshareable is received, deepening intersubjective capacity.

The Body Languaged by the Analysand

Direct body-based experience refers to what is happening in the moment in a bodily-felt way. Speaking in the first-person present tense brings this subjective reality alive in language. It also brings consciousness to bear on how such experience has, and is, an embodied psychic reality. Using the present tense lets the experience be lived in the saying rather than speaking of experience as something in the past. It also emphasizes the significance of the immediate implicit knowledge rather than situating it as an *aside* of less value to the content being spoken.

I echoed Róisín's words because I was sincerely moved and curious to know more. When Róisín expressed herself, and I responded in kind, the immediacy of the affect between us became alive, further "moving along" the interactive process where change occurs. What was voiced was a kind of call and response, calling forth more.[1]

I perceive the body's knowledge as a form of intelligence rather than solely as the repressed unconscious. I perceive change, in this context, as a moment of being *in* lived experience, which by its nature is transitory. The next moment is new and different. Being in the lived moment of affect, rather than talking about it, is, for me, like being immersed in the weather in the natural world. It is a moment-to-moment unfolding. Alive, changing. Moving on.

Summary

In this chapter, I have emphasized the importance of the therapist's and patient's use of language to reflect the embodied basis of the inner world and relationships. Most somatically based work focuses on grounding, regulation, flexibility, and integration. Most analytic work emphasizes the mind or minds of the analytic dyad with little attention to the body. Bringing the body into depth psychotherapy will always be entwined with affect and relationship, and with the relationship between the conscious and unconscious, the past, present, and prospective realms. Perhaps we can reach toward this more inclusive perspective in our language.

Note

1   Christopher Bollas (1987) describes echoing as a way to draw forth what (the unconscious) seeks to be known.

References

Abrams, D. (1996). *The spell of the sensuous: Perception and language in a more-than-human world* (pp. 45–46). New York: Pantheon Books.

Bollas, C. (1987). *The shadow of the object: Psychoanalysis of the unthought known.* London: Free Association Books.

Bruschweiler-Stern, N., Lyons-Ruth, K., Morgan, A. C., Nahum, J. P., & Reis, B. (2018). Moving through and being moved by: Embodiment in development and in the therapeutic relationship. *Psychoanalytic Inquiry, 38*(5), 311–326.

Bruschweiler-Stern, N., Lyons-Ruth, K., Morgan, A. C., Nahum, J. P., Sander, L. W., Stern, D. N., Harrison, A. M. & Tronick, E. Z. (2002). Explicating the implicit: The local level and the microprocess of change in the analytic situation. *International Journal of Psychoanalysis, 83*, 1051.

Fuchs, T. (2018). *Ecology of the brain.* Oxford: Oxford University Press.

Fuchs, T., & Koch, S. C. (2014). Embodied affectivity: On moving and being moved. *Frontiers in Psychology, 5*(508), 1–12.

Kalsched, D. (2013). *Trauma and the soul: A psycho-spiritual approach to human development and its interruption.* New York: Routledge.

Levine, P. A. (2010). *In an unspoken voice: How the body releases trauma and restores goodness.* Berkeley: North Atlantic Books.

Nye, N. S. (1998). *Fuel.* BOA Editions. www.boaeditions

Stern, D. N. (2010). *Forms of vitality: Exploring dynamic experience in psychology, the arts, psychotherapy, and development.* Oxford: Oxford University Press. https://doi.org/10.1093/med:psych/9780199586066.001.0001

Chapter 7

The Significance of the Body in Transforming Trauma from a Depth Psychotherapeutic Perspective

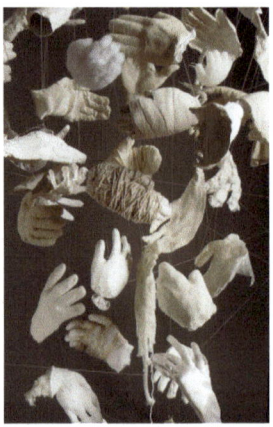

2nd Skin Detail (Rosalyn Driscoll, 2003–5, Steel, mixed media, 78" x 38" x 38". Photography by David Stansbury)

The emerging paradigm of working with trauma in psychoanalysis is increasingly more relational, understands the significance of attachment patterns, and is informed by infant studies, neuroscience, and trauma studies. In the preceding chapters, I have outlined the primal current of the experienced body in these realms. As we turn directly toward trauma, the bodily basis of experience is ever more significant. Much of the immediacy of trauma registers first bodily, then entwines with reflective processes of affect and cognition. This is true in early development and our earliest relationships as well. The body is a portal to access those direct experiences that are held in implicit relational memory, and revivified in the analytic dyad and the patient's outer life.

Working directly with the bodily basis of experience activates the inherent wisdom of our organism's capacity to co-regulate, self-regulate, and develop affect tolerance, creating fertile ground for new experiences to become available as the healing process unfolds. It adds dimensionality, grounds, and furthers the

DOI: 10.4324/9781003305804-8

possibilities of relationally based psychotherapeutic work. Yet, for these possibilities to be fully realized in the treatment of trauma, such an approach must recognize that

> *for every self–other relational moment in psychotherapy, there is also an inner event* and I don't mean an inner event in the wiring or sculpting of the brain. I mean an inner event in sculpting the soul—in what Jungians often call the ego–Self relationship or the ego–Self axis ... This space is "transitional," but not between self and other. Rather, this space is transitional between what James Grotstein (2000) calls the "ineffable subject of the unconsciousness" and the "phenomenal subject of consciousness".
>
> (Kalsched, 2013, p. 8)

With an often uncanny wisdom our dreams express this mythopoetic and sometimes numinous effect, as will be shown in the following case studies. When the dual vectors of bodily-based and mythopoetic experience are brought to consciousness, a very personally felt meaning unfolds and carries the work forward. Throughout his work, Jung emphasized psyche's innate thrust toward wholeness and the ideal of individuation. "But this ideal leaves out the agony of facing madness that has been eclipsed from our living" (Ulanov, 2020, p. 584). Facing the chaotic feelings dissociated in trauma is often messy work. For some, such as the two persons I will present in this chapter, working both vectors was essential to reclaiming the parts of the self that had been split off due to the unspeakable agony of traumatic experience. For one, trauma occurred well before words were acquired; for the other, a developmental traumatic incident momentarily extinguished consciousness. For both, memories of the traumatic events and the psychic agonies induced by them were imprinted in their bodies, and there they accrued archetypal elements that paradoxically protected the core self within yet inhibited the psyche's thrust toward wholeness (Kalsched, 2013).

The Imaginal Realm

Imaginal mythopoetic experience is an intermediary realm between the verbal and nonverbal and the visible and nonvisible worlds. Dreamwork, exploration of images, the Jungian process known as Active Imagination, artwork, affective responses, amplifications, and associations—all become avenues of its exploration. At times, the imaginal world offers a "*way in*" to the implicit unconscious; at times, contacting what lies in the somatic unconscious creates a bridge to consciousness and activates the psyche's symbolizing capacity. Sometimes, such a bridge is forged readily; sometimes, when trauma reigns, the bridge forms slowly through a process of titration—small moments strung together that bring coherence where fragmentation had reigned. But this is not a linear process, and it often leads both analysand and analyst to moments or periods of helplessness and exhaustion. Techniques and interpretations do not suffice in these spaces; the flickering candle in the dark becomes one's humanness, stripped down and dwelling with and through the not knowing (Cwik, 2011).

The Non-verbal Dimensions of the Numinous

When transformational moments do arise, the value of the numinous more fully emerges by slowing down and lingering in the nonverbal dimensions of those experiences. Entering such intimate and vulnerable territory with a patient expands the limits of what is shareable. Staying with the nonverbal experience allows it to be further known, deepening the felt experience of the patient and the analyst as well. In this way, a cellular imprint—a nondual reconfiguration of dynamic pathways— comes to indwell the psyche-soma. Jung spoke of how true transformation of the complex comes from an encounter with the numinous energies of the archetype— a truth even more significant in the fragmenting forces of trauma (1969/1954). When this happens, the body serves as a portal to the numinous dimensions of the soul's life—healing and wholeness that goes far beyond just the relief of traumatic symptoms, leading to increased access to feelings in general and a renewed sense of soulful aliveness.

Weaving an Approach to the Inner World of Trauma with the Polyvagal Theory of Emotion and Somatic Experiencing

While I draw from many sources when working with the inner world of trauma, Kalsched's model (2013) is a significant guide. When working with direct experience in the body, I draw from Peter Levine's Somatic Experiencing while incorporating Stephen Porges' polyvagal theory of emotion. I integrate these approaches in a relational, analytically oriented way.

I will give a brief overview of the polyvagal theory of emotion as I believe it both illuminates and can help guide our way when encountering what Kalsched refers to as archetypal affect indicative of trauma. I will also highlight aspects of Somatic Experiencing, which you will see come into play in the casework. Because the roots of unformulated experience dwell in the body, attending to somatic experience significantly augments our use of reverie and our understanding of unconscious communication.

A Depth Psychological Approach to the Inner World of Trauma and the Archetypal Self-Care System

In these troubled times, trauma is ubiquitous. It seems more and more patients present with complex trauma. As I write this chapter, war has broken out in the Middle East. The prevalence of war exponentiates the presence of trauma in the collective body across generations. In both of the cases I present in this chapter, the transgenerational transmission of trauma can be traced back to social and political conflict and war. Traumatic psychic structures give rise to polarizing attitudinal stances within the individual, manifesting in outer relationships with others. These inner–outer polarized positions can become entrenched as political ideologies. A psychological attitude to individual and group dynamics is essential if we wish to bridge the polarizations that divide our individual and collective body.[1]

In Kalsched's model of working with trauma, he likens the self-sabotaging defensive dynamic in the psyche to the fallen angel Dis, found in the depths of Hell in Dante's *Inferno* (Kalsched, 2013). Dis, who personifies the psyche's archetypal dissociative defenses, devours the innocent souls ensnarled in his underworld. *Dis* is derived from the Latin meaning to divide or negate. It is encountered clinically as dissociation, disavowal, dismissal, and disconnection. In his epic poem, Dante, amid a profound inner crisis, finds himself lost in this underworld realm that is lorded over by the personification of this dismembering daemon. Ultimately, guided by his companion, Virgil, they descend through the treacherous realms of endless suffering, at the frozen bottom of which the only way out is through an intimate encounter with the dark monster himself. This requires the pilgrim to muster every ounce of inner courage and to climb up the leg and groin of Dis to avoid his devouring grasp. In this manner, the pilgrim enters the realm where genuine suffering—experiencing feelings in the body—allows a passageway up and out into the bright, breathing world.

In Kalsched's formulation, the Self-care system comes into play as an attempt to protect the innocent core of the psyche, depicted as the soul–child, from ever having to bear again the highly charged archetypal affect that overwhelmed the psyche in trauma. With its benevolent, ideal, and spiritualized manifestation in the positive pole, or its devouring, negating, dismissive manifestation in the negative pole, the Self-care system's early intent to protect the innocent core of the psyche ultimately becomes entrapping. The traumatized person thus remains caught in an eternal struggle for redemption, a struggle for a sense of value and goodness. From an analytic perspective, we can envision this struggle as a yearning for a sense of undivided wholeness, the Self, that sacred sense of being in relation to the natural order of things, rather than shamefully cast out of the weave of belonging.

Embodied Self-protective Mechanisms

Exploring the embodied aspects of the psyche's self-protective mechanisms adds a palpable basis to the Self-care system (Kalsched, 1996, 2013). I believe this can aid the transformation of these tenacious dynamics. Having a felt sense of their physical manifestations provides a means to learn, from the body's wisdom, about their presence and function, giving rise to a deeper understanding and an appreciation of the genius of their role in an individual's survival. Sensing their postural expression and the embedded attitudes in these distinct parts of the inner world facilitates conscious, reflective dialogue between them. With that comes the possibility of purposefully releasing the embodied tensional patterns. Choice becomes available where there was none before. Changes in bodily-based experience in the service of linking to affect, memories, images, and meaning engage the whole person. This gives rise to new possibilities (Whitehouse, 2007).

In *Two Essays on Analytic Psychology* (1966/1943, p. 199), Jung reminds us that psychology is nothing if not experience. As I work with trauma, I return again and again to the felt experience of the breath in the body. Trauma restricts breath, deadening one's capacity to feel (Russell, 1999) and thus to engage with others with genuine rather than truncated emotional honesty. Awareness of the *sensory experience* of breathing illuminates *felt* experience. Doing so slows us down, aligning us with innate bodily rhythms. In an analysis, it can be the fertile moment in which past, present, and future come together in a still point of shared knowing.

The Polyvagal Theory of Emotion: the Neuropsychological Underpinnings of the Archetypal Affect Ignited in Trauma

I understand what Kalsched means when he uses *archetypal affect* in the context of trauma by weaving Jung's description of archetype as a psychic instinct with neuroscientist Stephen Porges' polyvagal theory of emotion (Porges, 2001). In brief, the *vagus* is a major nerve of the parasympathetic system, which functionally connects our brain to our body. It is a cranial nerve responsible for regulating internal organ functions, such as digestion, heart rate, and respiratory rate, as well as vasomotor activity and certain reflex actions, such as coughing, sneezing, swallowing, and vomiting. What is most important in thinking about the vagus is that it is not only a top-down but also a bottom-up nerve. Eighty percent of the fibers on the vagus are sensory. *The vagus is really our primary portal to brain–body and mind–body relationships* (Porges, 2001).

We have two types of vagi that evolved at different points. This is extremely important because the role each plays is quite distinct. The vagal pathways each come from two different areas of the brainstem. The evolutionarily newer one is unique to mammals. It plays a part in regulating and linking ingestion, the facial muscles we use to see, listen, and express our feelings to the other, and the heart—muscles activated in the primal act of nursing and throughout the life span as we engage others (Porges, 2009). "Our social nervous system is intimately related with this newer vagus—*and so is our breath*" (Porges, 2019, p. 4, italics added). Mammals "need other mammals to regulate their bodily states and to survive. ... *Trauma disrupts the ability to relate to others and to use social behavior to literally regulate vagal function—to calm us down*" (p. 4, italics added).

The second vagus extends below our diaphragm, regulating our viscera. We share this with many current vertebrates like reptiles and even fish. According to Porges, experiences of trauma overwhelm an individual's emotional coping capacity, activating a very primitive part of our organism, such that traumatic events are experienced as highly charged neurological arousal, or what I will call "instinctual arousal." I refer to this as instinctual arousal because the neurological system responds in a way that actually *precludes* felt emotion or cognition. The two neurological systems, the parasympathetic and the sympathetic, typically work harmoniously, enabling refined biological processes, "but they also react to the world—*we use them as defenses or responses to social challenges*" (2019, p. 5, italics added).

Porges distinguishes three basic neural subsystems that comprise the vagal nerve. With the help of Peter Levine's analysis of Porges, I describe how these kinds of vagal responses are based on the way an event is experienced.

Dissociation, Shutdown, Feigning Death, Freeze

If an event is perceived as physically life-threatening or psychologically threatening to one's very sense of self—with no potential for escape—a state of parasympathetic, hypo-arousal is activated, exerting the powerful effect of shutting down feeling and sensation and the capacity for thought—essentially a deadening or numbing. From an evolutionary perspective, this vagal subsystem originates in early fish and reptile species. The function of it is immobilization. Its target of action is the viscera—the immobilization of these leads to feigning death, shutdown, and dissociation (Levine, 2010).

Fight or Flee

If a threat is experienced with a sense that there is a chance to fight or flee, the sympathetic subsystem, which is next in evolutionary development and associated with the reptilian brain, is activated. This stimulates a release of adrenalin that increases heart rate, blood pressure, and breathing rate, inducing a state of highly charged hyper-arousal that activates the limbs.

Neuroception Is Well Below the Range of Consciousness: Biological Reactions Occur First

Both of these types of highly charged neural responses—dissociative shutdown and sympathetic hyper-arousal to fight or flee—*happen more quickly than cognition or emotional processes*. Porges refers to this unconscious evaluative process as "neuroception." *There is no conceptualization, emotion, or narrative unfolding.* Porges points out, "Neuroception is well below the range of consciousness ... *It is extremely important to understand this—the biological reaction occurs first*, and then we develop what I call personal narrative" (Porges, 2019, p. 9, italics added). In states of hypo-arousal, we shut down, play dead, or dissociate. In hyper-arousal, we become highly activated and charged to fight or flee. Often, there is a mixture of states.

The Social Engagement System

The third and most recent phylogenetic subsystem is activated when some potential for relational engagement is present. "This subsystem exists only in mammals and mediates attachment behaviors" (Levine, 2010, p. 99). Mammals are unique because they need other mammals to regulate their emotional and bodily states to survive. This is evident in our work as clinicians. However, when trauma occurs, and these more primitive systems take over the very possibility of relating to others, using social interaction to regulate vagal functioning—to calm us down—is disrupted, thus sabotaging us from getting that which we most need.

The Neurological Hierarchy of Default

Peter Levine describes this neurological hierarchy of default: if one perceives the environment as safe, one's social engagement system is activated. However, a less evolved system is engaged when pro-social behaviors do not resolve the threatening situation. We mobilize our fight-or-flight response. Finally, in this hierarchy of default, when neither of these more recently acquired systems (social engagement or fight/flight) resolves the situation, or when death appears imminent, the last-ditch system is engaged. This most primitive system, which governs immobility, shutdown, and dissociation, takes over and hijacks all survival efforts (Levine, 2010, pp. 99–100).

Story Making and Pre-Affective and Pre-Cognitive Events

These three states are pre-affective and pre-cognitive. Yet we are story-making creatures. Because we need a way to understand and make meaning of our experience, these inner states give rise to stories. However, this move into story or meaning often overrides the more instinctual dimensions. In bypassing the act of experiencing sensations, the discharge of the freeze response or sympathetic arousal is interrupted. The activated arousal remains in the body–mind—but is now disavowed or denied. This furthers a dissociative process. These residues accrue archetypal enhancements, and fortify identification with the attitudes of Dis, the archetypal dissociative force in the psyche (Kalsched, 2023, pp. 99–100, 116). Discerning what psychic attitudes shape inner stories is essential. It is counterproductive to align with the self-sabotaging forces in the psyche. Tracking the three kinds of vagal responses in my work with the women whose cases I present in this chapter was invaluable in sorting through their stories as we navigated the flow and counterflow of movement toward genuine embodied feeling.

An Overview of Important Concepts of Somatic Experiencing

Resourcing

Somatic Experiencing (SE) emphasizes "resourcing." Resourcing is the conscious recall or present-time experience of relating to or immersing oneself in things that nourish, soothe or inspire (Levine, 2010). This is frequently done at the start of an SE session. From an analytic perspective, I consider the analytic relationship to be the primary "resource." For me, it is the foundation of the analytic process. The notion of therapist as resource becomes quite complicated when the therapist is predominantly experienced as dangerous or untrustworthy in some way. I will describe such a situation as I carry forward my work with Eva, whom I spoke about in Chapter 2. In situations like these and many other instances, such as when the body itself is experienced as dangerous or plagued by symptoms and the source of misery, we may also focus on discovering "good" feelings in the body.

The Elements of Experience: Sensation, Images, Behavior, Affect and Meaning (SIBAM)

A fundamental principle of SE includes tracking the distinct elements that coalesce into internal experience. The acronym SIBAM stands for sensations, images, behavior, affect, and meaning, and aids in discerning the foreground element at play or absent. This can help guide engaging the patient in dialogue and refine interventions. For instance, in working with highly intuitive persons, what may be missing from their descriptions of experience are sensations and the direct experience of affect. Through attuned engagement, fostering awareness of these elements of the patient's experience can be extremely helpful in facilitating embodied, grounded experience. It also brings forth the immediacy of affect, linking these to memories (memories are incorporated into the umbrella of images in SIBAM) and other images, which are core to the healing of trauma.

Tracking the Meaning-Making Impulse

When working with the somatic unconscious in this way, it is often essential to refrain from jumping to meaning-making too soon. Humans, unlike animals, have such a strong propensity to cognitively override the bodily basis of the physiological aspects of traumatic experience and, by doing so, interrupt the capacity to feel. Because trauma is an injury in our capacity to feel (Russell, 1999), nothing could be more important than tracking this move to override or bypass. When direct experience is given its due, meaning often arises from the bottom up (the felt sense in the body) rather than needing to be overlayed by meaning that inadvertently overrides the body's knowing.

Sensations

Bringing felt experience to sensation occurring within, as well as to behaviors such as gestures, unconscious body movements, and patterns of holding, are often the portal into directly experiencing the body. Developing the capacity to sense, feel, and track unfolding sensations is revolutionary in psychotherapy, bringing an added dimension to the entirety of the process. The careful tracking of unfolding experience contributes to the regulation of hyper- and hypo-arousal, allowing affects to begin to emerge and take form, be felt, and find meaning.

Titration

Trauma occurs when a person encounters more feelings and sensations than can be borne. When this occurs, such an event is *felt* as threatening, sometimes life-threatening. The organism experiences overwhelm. Thus, in the work of healing trauma, the orientation is to titrate the hyper- or hypo-arousal bit by bit so as not to retraumatize the individual. This marks the difference between this approach and those that seek healing through catharsis. In this approach, work occurs gradually as all the elements of experience are integrated and embodied. In this way, working with the bodily aspects of experience can, without too much difficulty, easily fit into an analytic approach. The following cases will demonstrate this and the other principles discussed.

Pendulation

Traumatic residues have the propensity to haunt a person. One of the cornerstones of working with the bodily basis of trauma, giving a further dimension to Jung's concept of the transcendent function, is bearing the tension of opposite pulls in the psyche in an embodied way to allow a third thing to emerge. Peter Levine engages polarized states in the body in a process he calls "pendulation" (2010). The therapist might facilitate this process when a person is caught in what he calls a traumatic vortex—especially when dissociation, collapse, and depersonalization are active. Pendulation is also useful when a person is highjacked by the reptilian brain's response to fight or flee. When working with the body in movement with the transcendent function, the Jungian analyst, Joan Chodorow (1999/1978) cogently describes the value of experiencing the transcendent function in the body. She tracks how a person experiences sensations of constriction as arising from the somatic unconscious. As awareness of sensations becomes conscious, that awareness unfolds in the body. The body now becomes the seat of consciousness. The act of sensing creates proprioceptive feedback, which confronts the unconscious with the body ego's reality. "Since the body has the capacity to simultaneously manifest both conscious and unconscious, it may be our most potent tool toward the transcendent function" (p. 247).

Savoring experiences valued as "good" in the body consciously is particularly useful to those who have suffered trauma. Doing so helps lay down new neural networks, shifting attention from an over-focus on feelings, thoughts, and ruminations shrouded in a negative valence.

Orienting

When necessary, shifting attention to elements in the room, such as the therapist's Presence or voice, the natural world, and beyond also shifts a neurologically wired traumatic orientation to a wider, more flexible one. In Somatic Experiencing, this is referred to as orienting. When one purposefully focuses on elements in the environment by turning their head *and* neck and, if possible, the whole spinal column so to engage the deep vagal nerve, the outer world can again be seen and sensed shifting the neurological "freeze" or fixation of trauma. It is what animals do once they feel the threat has passed to assure themselves of that safety. Humans can cognitively override this step by dismissing, denying the impact of trauma, moving on before their organism has had time to reorganize to a sense of safety.[2]

Case Studies

While many of the vignettes introduced throughout this book point to how developmental trauma registers in the body, this chapter focuses specifically on the complex bodily basis of traumatic experience and the psyche's unfolding response to that wounding and its healing. These traumatic sequelae underscore the need to closely attend to somatic experience, allowing affects-in-the-body to emerge and formulate into conscious awareness. The following case studies illuminate how the mythopoetic realities revealed in that therapeutic process weave a tapestry of personal meaning, facilitating integral psychological–soulful transformation.

Turning an inward eye to healing trauma, Kalsched reminds us that

> to carry something consciously is not just a matter of adjusting our mental attitudes or of insight alone: the great *coniunctio* that we're after with these patients—and that Jung discussed in reference to the dis-embodied "opposites"—cannot happen without the body and its unredeemed, unknown, un-remembered, and frozen affects. In trying to heal our capacity to feel, we're pursuing a consciousness of the heart. That, for me, is the numinous *mysterium* in what Jung (1963) called the *Mysterium Coniunctionis*. The heart is the hidden third. And recovering a heart that can break is how we help ourselves and our patients recover the capacity to feel.
>
> (Kalsched, 2020, p. 149)

The Case of Eva (continued from Chapter 2)

Finding, Touching, and Feeling Her Hidden Heart

Eva, whom I introduced in Chapter 2, came into the session struggling to work through the upset that arose when she and her daughter clashed around the COVID-19 vaccine. Eva struggled to allow her daughter, in her early twenties, to have her own thoughts and feelings alongside Eva standing firm in her own. Not only does Eva have health conditions that put her at risk, but she was also concerned that exposure to COVID-19 would force her either to isolate or risk exposing friends and colleagues. Her daughter, who also has complex medical issues, had just returned from an extended time away. She had gone unvaccinated to a large political event in which many shared her distrust of the vaccine. Eva wanted her to take a COVID test before returning home, which her daughter strongly opposed. Eva's concerns for her daughter extended beyond the immediate vaccine issue, to her exposure to worldviews embedded in morals and values that did not sit well with Eva.

Eva became agitated as she described her dilemma to me. The difficult feelings she was encountering included the fear that I might judge her parenting. It was hard for her to stay focused. She veered into other dilemmas. She became increasingly riled up, and no intervention I tried—attunement, empathy, reflection, interpretation, or simply asking if she could slow down—shifted her delivery. She continued, talking over me but a bit louder. I was feeling very ineffectual and found it hard to stay with her. I found myself inwardly bracing. Rather desperately she told me she didn't want to be caught up in agitation like this. I noticed she was making a gesture—her arms extended out to the sides of her body, rotating around and around.

I ask, "Perhaps you can notice the gesture you are making—I hear you say you don't want this—to be caught up in this agitated state. I wonder what it would be like if you tried reversing the gesture?"

She tells me she cannot remember what she was doing—what direction her arms were moving. I suggest that rather than being concerned about exactly what gesture she had been making, she simply allows a gesture to arise that "feels" to be the opposite of what she had been doing. She extends her arms, then brings them over her head, brings them together, and slowly lowers them down along the center of her torso. This has an immediate effect.

She says, "Wow, that's amazing. I feel completely different. Like that settled the stirred-up muddy pond. My arms are tingling—like joy."

I am as surprised as she is about the radical change. I invite her to feel the sensations and, if she wants, to explore the gesture again. She does and reports a deepening sense of grounding and calming. She excitedly exclaims that she could do this when she has social anxiety!

Eva asks, "Is this what you call the transcendent function?"[3]

I respond encouragingly, but I do not want to get too conceptual. I suggest we stay with her felt sense a bit longer before we talk about it. I invite her to return to her experience and notice what she feels in her lower belly, center, and legs as she gestures.

She says, "Being in my body—I guess that's the key, isn't it? I guess I caved with the COVID test. I got all goofy when I tried standing up for myself. It's like I'm not worthy of saying No." She says she can hear the little girl in her voice.

I ask, "What was it like to stand up for yourself as a little girl."

Eva replied, "Oh, my father would just yell or something. But with my mother—I guess I never did. It was better not to—not to have an accident."

I notice a wave of anxiety in my core and chest.

Eva says, "When I do it now—stand up for myself—I feel all tense. A jumble in my chest."

I say, "That little girl in you sacrificed a lot."

The comment helps bring her back into a symbolizing adult part of herself, recognizable by a change in her voice. I ask what she would like that little girl to know now.

Eva says, "That it was not her fault. I thought I wasn't worthy of saying No."

She associates this with Thích Nhất Hạnh,[4] recalling how he does that with dignity. We acknowledge that he, too, had been through a war.

With curiosity, we continue to explore the effect the gesture has on her internal state. She speaks of the repetitious pull to take care of others, and how the gesture opens the potential for the opposite: to take care of herself. It allows her to come back into herself after having abandoned herself. Both gestures, held consciously, activated the transcendent function, bringing forth an affective, embodied transformation.

The arising of the gesture is important not only to the moment at hand but also regarding healing her trauma. She has practiced *Qi Gong* and *Tai Chi*, but ultimately, the intense internal pressures to be good, coupled with inner criticism, undermined these from feeling sourced from within. They became yet another thing she was not doing "right." The spontaneous arising of the gesture locates its authenticity squarely in herself. This is an important part of furthering her work of embodiment. Later, we discuss how her gesture has archetypal roots in the ancient practice of *Qi Gong*. It facilitates grounding and centering one's core source of power in resonance with the natural world.[5]

Having a need that Eva perceives as conflicting with another's stirs a traumatic, implicit, body-based, relational memory—she dissociates from her need, abandoning herself. When in this state, she completely cuts off from her body and has no awareness of feelings. In the arms of the bright angel of the Self-care system, she becomes the "good" girl, and care takes the other. This also assures her some sense of connection. Having worked in this territory before, she can sometimes re-center to a less polarized position. Right now, she continues to feel moved by how the calmness that emerged as she gestured stays with her.

The slow titration of this and other traumatic responses we have worked on laid the groundwork for the restoration of a cohesive sense of self (coherent ego function). The somatic work has helped to restore her interoceptive awareness. The spontaneous arising of the gesture opened the possibility to not just reflect but to experience a new embodied attitude—a third position arose that led to impulses finding containment, polarization being buffered, and the new experience lived. From this lived experience came the possibility of inner coherence and reflection (Stein, 1998, p. 124). Research has shown impaired processing of interoceptive signals in states characterized by emotional dysregulation (Paulus & Stein, 2010; Herbert, Herbert & Pollatos, 2011; Muller et al., 2015). The gesture allowed interoceptive awareness to develop and with this came emotional coherence and differentiation.

Eva created Figure 7.1 to depict her experience of the little girl whose voice is frozen by the persecuting force of the Self-care system that demands the disavowal of feelings. The other protecting pole of the Self-care system swoops her up into

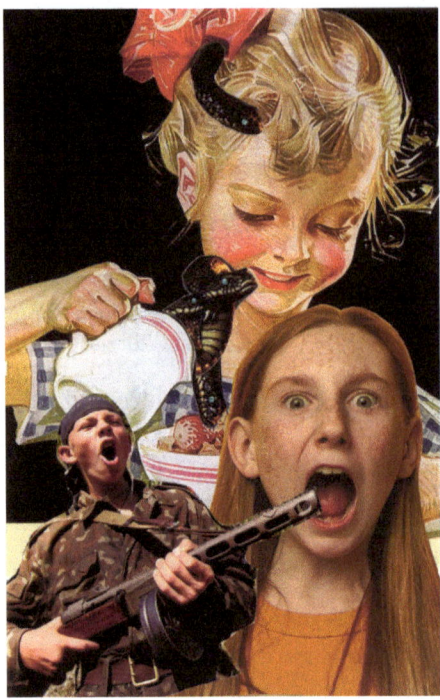

Figure 7.1 Young girl caught between the positive and negative sides of the Self-care system (Original artwork by Eva, with permission)

the mesmerizing promise of being "good." However, snakes pour forth from the milk, depicting the good girl's terror that any moment, if an "accident" were to occur, she could be attacked and have her hair pulled out, as her mother would sometimes do. This terror overshadows any other feelings she might have, including rage about the relentless demand to be good.

A Dream Emerges Following Her Gesture

She brings this dream to the next session:

> *I am in this class with a movement teacher. I am doing something with my arm, moving it really slowly (Eva gestures, her arm bent at the elbow, her hand and upper arms sweep slowly from left to right, level with her chest).*
>
> *In the dream, I got it ... to be in my body brings not just a sense of presence, but more FEELING. I was so pleased!*

Then the teacher gave me another thing to do, almost a cognitive test, like a SAT, the opposite of a Jungian way, more like the Guttenberg way (Guttenberg is her last name, and an oft-repeated repetitive family saying is: 'You are a Guttenberg!' meaning you will earn a Pulitzer Prize—as her aunt had).

Now, in the dream, we are on a break from the class. The teacher's husband is there and is acting competitively, wanting to impart his wisdom.

She says she understands that in the dream, the husband is herself, an animus figure (or the dark angel Dis)—that cuts her off from feeling. Then, she shifts to the present and reports being physically cold. The session is on Zoom, and the place she goes to do this is not always comfortable.

However, she goes on to say, "Maybe I freeze inside. I think I don't feel connected unless you are really happy with me. I feel this tension in my chest. I am waiting to see if you are happy with me."

I say, "The tension really keeps you on guard."

Eva stays with the felt sense of the freeze and accompanying vigilance. She senses the gripping in her chest that constricts her breathing so she can't feel much else. The gripping lessens somewhat, and her breath comes in with more fullness, followed by a big exhale.

She says, "I want to get back to that ah-ha feeling place."

She tells me how she feels loss and despair at losing contact with where she had been. She then expresses this sense of the dream—that this beauty came forth—when she was in a group moving together.

She says, "But it is tense for me if I don't know whether you are happy with me."

I softly echo her.

Eva says, "Yeah, earlier, I got anxious. I just want to get back—when I get cognitive, I go away from the slow, feeling place."

Both of us are bringing more empathy to the inner conflicts that are rooted in the accommodations she constantly made when with her mother in an attempt to not trigger an attack. Now, with her daughter's unique needs, this old pattern of behavior is revivified and further complicated by her concern that I don't approve of her. I easily empathize with how frightened she becomes, and understand how this interferes with her desire to stand up for her own needs now. It is important to remember that for that little girl within, her mother's attacks felt life-threatening—and whatever she could do to help her feel safe in those times was paramount (Bromberg, 2011, p. 23). She exhales audibly and lets down some of her vigilance with me.

By weaving the work with her dreams, memories, artwork, and our relationship with ongoing attention to the bodily-based felt sense of the vigilance and traumatic freeze response, we titrate the traumatically charged affect bit by bit. After each round, a deeper layer of pain or longing emerges to be addressed.

She tells me her first dream of last night:

> *She "got" that my name was Barbara—you are not just my therapist—you are a real person with a name. She says: I hadn't really gotten that before.*
> *She associates back to the dream she first told me.*
> *And says, "My strongest feeling in that dream is when the teacher stopped me from feeling."*

I am left wondering if I was represented in the dream as the teacher and how I might have stopped her from feeling in that last session and if we can talk about that before moving to this new dream. But before I say anything, she jumps in with a story about a client of hers and his obsessional tendencies, adding that his daughter committed suicide.

I empathically respond to what she has just said, "just scary … and painful."

She cuts me off and, with a gesture, says: "OFF WITH YOUR HEAD! You are Bad, that's it!"

I understand she is expressing the inner voice of the negative Self-care system, chopping off our attention to these emerging tender parts of her. The protective mechanism doubles down when feelings start to emerge—the affects are barely tolerable, and this is creating a tumble inside.

> *Spontaneously, she returns to the gesture in the dream—enters it again—and surprisingly finds that now, it stirs an intense tingling in her arms.*
> *She pauses to feel this and then says, "It's a spiritual thing like meta/love."*
> *She repeats: "Oh, if I go slow, I have feelings."*

I understand her to be expressing that her heart softens when she feels safe, though I don't say this. We both continue to be taken by the effect of the gesture. It lessens the hyperactivation she experiences, allows for more affect tolerance, and helps reinstate cognitive organization.

Eva soon says, "But then I lost it in the dream. Maybe I am afraid I will lose it forever."

I reflect aloud, "That is what it feels like—when you are cut off from your feelings, they just seem gone. But today, you didn't forget forever; you remembered and returned to that part of you that wants to feel and has feelings.

Perhaps I did not bring words to the possibility that maybe she had feelings of love for me, fearing it would be just too vulnerable. For instance, whenever I ask how it will be for her when I am on vacation, she quickly replies, "I don't feel anything." Yet, nevertheless, when she re-entered the gesture, it stirred her deeply and unexpectedly. Her words, "It's a spiritual thing like meta/love," and the way she spoke them, conveyed that.

Figure 7.2 emerged sometime after this session. In the far upper right is a newborn, immersed in a confusing blur, blocking anyone outside her from getting too close. On the left, the hand that reaches to touch another. The image has a similar theme and feel to Michelangelo's painting on the ceiling of the Sistine Chapel, which Kalsched uses to exemplify the divine union with one's united self, experienced when the vulnerable inner soul–child is liberated from the grips of the dark and light angels of the Self-care system. In Eva's artwork, a butterfly in the center appears, symbolizing release from those constricting binds. Though incredibly vulnerable, she is daring to make a voluntary sacrifice of the "cocoon" of self-sufficiency for the safety of our therapeutic relationship (Modell, 1993). Ursula Wirtz (2021/2014, p. 291) reminds us that such a voluntary sacrifice can be an antidote to the traumatic involuntary sacrifice that was required by Eva when her psyche recruited the Self-care system rather than suffer psychic annihilation. This inner self-protective cocoon preserved her spark of divine innocence within.

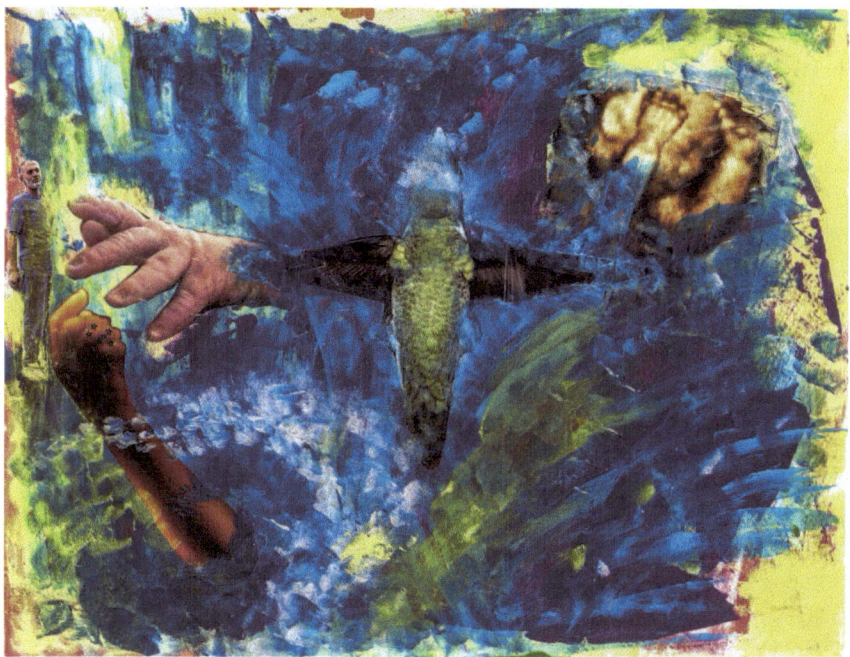

Figure 7.2 Distressed infant in fetal position and the wounded child within now reaching for connection (Original artwork by Eva, with permission)

Dis Doubles Down: Enactments Unfold

Loosening the grips of the Self-care system she was able to feel more into the sense of chaos and psychophysical disorganization. She depicted this experience in her artwork and brought it in to show me (not depicted here). In this piece, a girl–woman is caught in a dark blue, swirling realm cluttered with bits of hair and other debris. There is no one in the picture but her. She feels alone in the midst of confusion. She felt this vulnerability as she created the artwork, and also as we explored her feelings and associations arising when she brought it into her session. The psychic space between us opened. We were relating in a more intersubjective way.

From a perspective informed by Somatic Experiencing, the hyper-arousal Eva experiences is being titrated, allowing the social engagement system to activate. Not infrequently, this enables yet another layer of traumatic psychophysically charged pain to arise and be titrated, which is what follows.

Eva goes on to tell me about a dilemma in which colleagues asked her to bring some food for an event, and she said yes, even though she did not really want to. She was afraid of being seen as not altruistic. Because she will need to prepare food for the event and is insecure about her cooking, she chooses to bring a dish in at the end of the week in hopes that this will give her plenty of time. However, the task loomed in her mind and she found herself ruminating about what needed to be done and what might go wrong.

She says, "Just thinking about it gives me this feeling of anxiousness in my arms. Accidents, I can't predict the outcome. It makes me anxious in my lower arms and chest."

Without understanding what is suddenly occurring, we both get swept up in a psychic swirl (as portrayed in her artwork not shown here—a girl in the center of a dark, circling swoon of bits of pulled-out hair and other debris). I began to feel intensely hyper-aroused and realized an enactment was occurring, but I could not get a conscious sense of what was unfolding.

As she talks, she corrects me when I fail to reflect her words accurately. She continues in an agitated way, and I continue to miss getting it right, which makes her more anxious. She tries to get me to match her—I am not able to. It becomes unbearable (to her, to me—and, it seems, to us both). This registers in me as both physical turmoil in my guts and emotional overwhelm such that I am unable to think or feel with any clarity. When I manage to say something, she responds, "What are we talking about? are we talking about, shame—me being a bad person?"

While these words Eva has just spoken do seem to get straight to the point, in the moment, nothing seemed particularly clear to me except that we had entered territory characterized by disorganization and dissociation.

In reflection, I wonder if it is as if I am, at that moment, like her mother, not able to match/attune to her. If she is not able to get me to do what she needs, then fear of her mother's possible reaction sets in, leading to an inner state of disorganization and then dissociation. What she is left with in her awareness is her default assessment that it is her fault—she is bad and shameful.

I want to help her find a way to buffer the intensity of her experience of shame. Bromberg (2011, p. 23) emphasizes the importance of addressing the shame evoked in the therapeutic process of reliving trauma in a relational context, referencing Lynd's (1958, p. 42) understanding of shame:

> Because of the outwardly small occasion that has precipitated shame, the intense emotion seems inappropriate, incongruous, disproportionate to the incident that has aroused it. *Hence a double shame is involved*; we are ashamed because of the original episode and ashamed, because we feel so deeply about something so slight that a sensible person would not pay any attention to it.
>
> (Lynd in Bromberg, 2011, p. 23, original emphasis)

I suggest that perhaps it is not so helpful to label her experience of herself here but, instead, to try to just be with it. Slowly, we reflect on how she had recounted an anxious feeling in her arms and chest when faced with the unpredictable situation with her colleagues. Additionally, she feared that I might judge her feelings and behavior. Because of all of this, she pressures herself to be *good and do it right* because if she can do it right, it binds the terrible feeling. And then she can hope that she will be seen in a favorable way. But sadly, this worsens it.

What I meant in that cryptic comment was that it binds her fear—with hopes that she will not encounter the possibility of the terrible storm of fear and terror—what Bromberg calls the "shadow of the tsunami" (2011, pp. 4–5). It is the terror she feels if someone sees her as bad—because in the past, at its worst, her mother could attack her if she did it wrong. When this happened, Eva would feel that it wasn't simply that what she had done was bad, but that she herself was bad and shameful.

Eva asks, "How does my trying to be good make it worse?"

I answer, "Because though you volunteered to help (to be seen as good), you put it off with hopes that doing so would free you from the terrible anticipation of it going wrong, but you got caught up in a kind of automatic thinking about it——and that kind of thinking, over and over—confirms that you are bad."

She reflects on this a bit. Then, she lapses into stories about her father not being able to help her and her memory of feeling afraid—that no one could help her.

I'd like to acknowledge and empathize with how unprotected she was (Davies & Frawley, 1994, p. 168),[6] but she interrupts, talking in an increasingly agitated and loud way. She raises her voice to control my response and keep back the flood and confusion of traumatic affect—I am more an object now than a person with a name whom she can relate to in an intersubjective way. A sense of safety between us is not accessible. Simultaneously, it seems to me as if, now, I have taken on Eva's position with her mom. I experience Eva's voice ever louder and more piercing. The piercing goes straight through me and feels awful. I think/feel her behavior is like her mother's, not in content, but in process.

From a state of something like desperation, I say something like, "This has to end—I cannot continue with this. This is not good for me. And I don't imagine it is good for you or your therapy."

We are both a bit stunned. As we reflect on what has happened, we are able to talk about my setting a limit to her talking over me with such a raised voice. She understandably becomes frightened that I am ending the therapy with her.

I say, "No, I am not. As we continue our work, you will certainly feel a need to protest. However, I need you to be willing to actively participate in reflecting on the impulse and begin to slow down and pause and sense how you are affecting me."

She is concerned that she will have to be perfect, or I will end the therapy. I acknowledge her fear yet wonder aloud that if she pauses and thinks about it, perhaps in actuality, there might be *more room* to find clarity and thus more possibility for truly feeling her feelings rather than just her raw reactions. Maybe we would be able to reflect on them together.

One part of her gets it. But another part breaks in—she becomes the three-year-old in voice and body (swinging her legs, with a young, high-pitched voice) filled with fear that she has to do it right, be good, or she is afraid I will end the therapy—abandon her).

I recount how I know she values her work in therapy and wants to continue, and I let her know I want to continue with her. I reflect on how when she is really afraid, the scared little girl takes over. I ask if she can take a moment to remember if, in our work, she has felt there is room for her feelings with me over the years. This helps her shift to an adult self-state, capable of symbolic reflection.

She says she has. We are able to end the session in a more related way, albeit shakily.

Discovering Limit Setting Through an Enactment

She begins the following session by recounting a time years ago when she was in a group at Mt. Shasta. They were doing a quest. Each of them was in a designated place, alone on the mountain. She shared how, in a moment in which she felt the depth of her despair about ever being able to take in the love she longed for, her longing became a heartfelt prayer. It was then that she saw a glimmering off on the distant slope. She went there and found it was an old, weathered bible. She opened to a passage that read: "Ask, and it will be given to you; seek, and you will find; knock, and it will be opened to you."

She says it was amazing and synchronistic, and even though that happened, she throws her spiritual experiences in the garbage. She recounts how once, while doing a walking meditation on a day-long retreat, she intentionally walked toward a trash can—which represented her desire to look at her own inner garbage. There, she found a pearl next to the trash can. For her, it confirmed her intention to continue with her inner work—"Like I keep getting the message but don't receive it."

She explains how she had imagined that if she collected enough such synchronistic events, it would be proof that she was worthy. She is so disappointed with herself because she is not able to hold the memory of these events inside—she quickly loses track of them (dissociates). But she is now coming to understand that the value is not about accumulating synchronistic events but about internalizing a feeling of self-worth. When we are together, she can feel and remember that she *is* doing the work with her traumatic past that is necessary for that internalization to occur. In other words, she is finding access to that treasure hard to attain—the pearl found amidst the trash and the rubble—her feeling heart.

Her inability to sustain a sense of her inner value is rooted in early experiences in which her mother and father failed to convince her of the genuine love they felt for her as a person—as opposed to their need for her to be good or their idealized expectation of her achieving fame. Caught in the midst of this dynamic, she withdrew her feelings of vulnerability and presented a false self—a part of her that engaged the external world with some sense of security. However, when she is caught in the complexity of this trauma dynamic, though she exhibits some sense of security, inwardly, she doubts herself and doubts that what she does matters (Kalsched, 2013, pp. 106–107).

I ask her, "What about here with me? Do you sense that I value you?"

We talk about our last session. She felt I was really mad. I let her know that, actually, I was hurting.

Very surprised, she says, "When you said 'I don't think this is good for me,' I thought you meant your nervous system."

I let her know that I am a whole person and that she was right; it had gone straight through to my nervous system, which felt alarming. I knew it needed to stop. That is what registered first, then later, because I am a whole person, not just a nervous system; I could recognize that I felt hurt like I had been violated or run over, disrespected.

In an arrested way, she apologizes and softens, letting me know she had not known that. And quickly adds, "You seemed angry. You said you were frustrated."

I suggest we slow down our interchange, that a lot happened in a very short time, and that there is value in talking about it carefully. As we both re-entered with a bit more cautious curiosity, I let her know that I had felt frustrated and then alarmed. I wondered aloud (as it was just occurring to me) if perhaps I was able to set a limit in a way that she had never been able to do with her mother when she was a child because it was so scary and she was so little.

She jumps in, letting me know that she had just been thinking that—but had not wanted to talk over me or interrupt. We pause, lighter in feeling now, knowing we'd both had the same thought somewhat simultaneously. I wonder aloud if, in the enactment, some part of her (though not consciously) was trying the best way she knew to let me know what it was like to be with her mom when her mom was attacking her. She lets this in. I say, "It seems like it was overwhelming—just how awful and scary *it was*."

As we further reflect on what happened, neither of us can remember the content of what we had been talking about during that session before the tumult. I say aloud that it is okay that in an enactment like the one we fell into, it is likely more about the process than the content (she has some understanding of this term because she is a therapist). I explain a bit more, letting her know that an enactment is something like both our unconscious processes being thrown together and what arises is something like a dream—though a waking dream. If we can reflect on it, like we might on a dream, it might offer us something more than we were able to get at consciously.

The pause opens reflective space and we try to piece together what had happened. I comment on how the good-girl part of her gets scared and second-guesses what she thinks I am going to say, and speaks this before I speak, throwing us out of relationship. When I try to slow us down, and she talks over me, it further breaks our connection. She agrees. I comment on how we are relating just now; it feels different, yet it is not effortful.

She agrees. She softens. She tells me how, at the clinic where she works, if a client is aggressive or attacking and demanding, she tries to stay with them, but in doing so, they aren't really engaged in dialogue. Her sessions with them become difficult—less related—and it is harder to stay present or feel their progress. Eva tells me very sincerely how she appreciates that I keep trying to find her and recognize the defenses as distinct from her person.

I spontaneously let her know I think she is a gem. And I find it easy to like and enjoy her. I appreciate how crucial those self-protective mechanisms were in her early life, but now they break our capacity to relate, and that saddens me. She lets me know she feels reassured.

In our discussion, we pieced the enactment together in a more linear way than it occurred. It was nonlinear, and we were both shifting identifications. The session ends.

Next Session

She tells me she'd been really scared last session. Then she adds, "But then we got through it." She says very relatedly, "You raised the bar (of our work, my therapy)." She speaks of how she loves it when, in a session, she shifts to a part of her that can feel. She experiences this as confirmation that she is really doing therapy (rather than spinning in the vortex of traumatic defenses).

Not only did she express her feelings in this session, but we also began to interact in a more related way. Most frequently, I serve a self-object function for her. Her earlier dream depicted me as a real person, evident by her learning I have a name. I am not an object that serves her needs and has no feelings. I am someone who can be hurt (as was she in childhood, though this was never acknowledged by her mother). Feeling this, she moves into the depressive position—where interpersonal relating is possible (Segal, 1973). She finds herself to be a person who feels sad for hurting another.

That dream, like others, shapes her inner experience into a narrative that arises from within her, and the feeling and meaning of it can linger inside as this new reality takes root. I perceive her dream arising from the part of her expressing this urge to grow and to truly relate by feeling—the ego–Self axis is restored in finding she has feelings for another (Kalsched, 2013, p. 107).

Eva's Anger Takes Form

Having worked through this important territory, something shifted in the following session; she reported having felt unseen by me. Feeling angry, she stood up to me, telling me she wanted what I suggested was missing. We both agreed that bringing even a little conscious reflection to bear on the moments of dissociated talk was needed. However, she was angry that I thought she was unaware of wanting that.

A dream soon followed: the foreign "not me" part of herself was depicted as rambunctious little boys creating mayhem inside a house. This was pivotal in marking a shift in her work. As we worked with it, the protesting part of her ultimately found a symbolic gesture. She imagined a gesture that flung the coveted yet dreaded tea across my office, which was a way of saying "No"—I am not going to be trapped by this demand that I never make a mistake, that I always be good, "No," I will not be held prisoner, will not be chained to this demand any longer. In protest, she proclaimed: I am a person, not a prisoner or the bad child of the dark angel or the "good" child of the bright angel in some imagined universe; I am a person with strengths and foibles.

Opening the Frozen Heart by Bringing Consciousness to an Enactment

In a session not too long after this, we fall into "it" again. She feels I do not get her, and falls into what I experience as a long, recounting of what is happening. Again, no matter how I try to intervene, which I believe, in my frustration, was less than skillful, and acknowledge what I had said that did not land well with her, she does not pause to hear me. Though I try in various ways to acknowledge my part, she persists.

I suddenly feel incredibly agitated inside. I try to enlist her in curiosity about what is happening between us. She tells me she doesn't know why I am so upset, and that she is trying to calm me down. Because this has happened before, it is more familiar. However, again, I do not really know what is happening; I do know I feel very dysregulated. I strive to bring consciousness to what is happening in me, but it is very hard to find any clarity. Again, I try to enlist her in being curious about what is happening between us. Acknowledging that, yes, I am feeling impatient and agitated.

At some point, somewhat desperate, I asked, "Was your mom impatient?"

She says, "My dad was. My mom was just intolerant."

Eva suddenly jumps in and says, "Let's start over. What should we talk about?"

I wonder aloud if this is a bit like what her mother would do after she would erupt at Eva. In the past, she has told me that after an explosion, her mother would later ask her in a sing-song voice if she wanted some "chicky"— a familiar food they would eat together. This is how they would continue together, but there was never repair or acknowledgment, so there was never true relating. She agrees that yes, maybe it was.

Spontaneously, she does the gesture of several sessions ago—extending her arms, sweeping them up over her head and with palms open and facing down, slowly lowering them down the length of her torso, following the energy and feeling the sensations of it traveling through her core. Immediately, her hyper-arousal down-regulates.

I find a way to inwardly surrender my urge to remain separate and instead join with her.

We are moving in synchrony. There is a calming, playful quality to this. She is smiling, happy, relieved. She then announces that this is the first time she has seen a woman go from being crazy to calm. She speaks of how we connected, and it was fun. As a way through enactments to new relational possibilities and psychic restructurings, Ringstrom says, "By humanizing the dyad's engagement, improvisational moments facilitate the dyad's connection amidst its necessary faltering when confusion, uncertainty, deadness, detachment, avoidance, or frightening combat must hold sway" (2007, p. 94).

My reverie drifts to what she told me about how, when she was young and with her friends, she would stay back and only join with them after observing for a time. I also recall Eva's mother told her when Eva was maybe three years old that she had found her hitting her doll. This went on for many days. Her mother told her she just couldn't stand seeing this, so she gave the doll away to a thrift store. Her mother said that Eva had cried and cried. Eva's mother's first hospitalization occurred when Eva was three years old. Later, when Eva was training to be a therapist, she realized the significance of her "play" and how some possibility for healing had been silenced at that time. We have found a way to play in our work together—such as joining in this gesture. At times, we can also symbolically "play" with her dreams and artwork.

She recounts how being left alone as a child after the incidents of her mom terrorizing her were so hard. Nodding, I said, something happened between us today.

She tells her young self, "You are not bad." Still processing, she again comments on how it feels we have raised the bar in her therapy—but it is scary for her when I am acting crazy. We reviewed the experience of making the gesture together and how she wanted me to join her, and she was glad when I did. This has a happy emotional tone to it. It seems she has enlisted me in a repair. It was empowering for her and deeply relieving.

Inwardly, I reflect on Bromberg's (2011) notion that therapy must provide safety and risk, especially if the analytic dyad is to tolerate and work through enactments. He stresses that the primary orientation is for the patient to know that the analyst is attuned to their affective well-being.

She continues processing, "Coming into this world is fragile and edgy, like walking across a war field. They didn't remove the mines."

We reflect on the terrible conflict she faced when she was very young. She needed her mother, needed to eat, and her mom could be so terribly scary. We reflect on the decision she told me she had made: not to need or cry. For a few minutes, we jointly empathize with that young part of her, feeling and understanding what an impossible situation that was. She points to the image of the bloody baby nursing from the breast of Medusa, which she has laid out on the floor between us (Figure 2.1).

She jumps in to let me know, again, that her mother was sad to stop nursing her when she was three months old. The doctor advised her mother to stop nursing because she had gotten a virus.

Eva says, "You think I am protecting her."

I respond, "No, that was the complexity you had to struggle with; your mom loved you—and she would lose it."

Eva says, "Yeah, I guess I can imagine that if poop leaked or I threw up or spit up all over, she'd screech. When she screeched, it was so loud and awful."

I respond with an attuned grimace and ask what it is like for her inside as she talks about it now—she was so little then, and the screeches were so upsetting.

She says, "I feel it in my heart."

I asked her what it was like there.

She says, "My breath is short, scared, and … paralyzed a bit."

We have entered the deep shutdown/freeze around her heart pertaining to her capacity to feel.

I sigh responsively, and we linger there; in time, I ask if it would feel ok for her to bring her hand to that part of her. She puts her hand on her heart.

With the prosody of my voice matching the relational moment, I say, "Yeah, just being with that part that got so scared and a little paralyzed." I hear a small inhalation and see her body begin to settle—to let down the tensional forces of the freeze of her heart.

She tells me that the little girl is a part she talks to sometimes. And it is the little girl who often just starts talking when in session with me. She says she sometimes talks to the little girl when she is alone in the car. And the little girl talks to her. She says it is almost like a separate part of her. She had not realized how the dissociative processes that had saved her had also fragmented her, leaving such a schism within.

I am relieved to hear her give voice to this. From the start of our work, it was apparent that Eva's self-states shifted rapidly. Most frequently, the terrified little girl, possessed by the inner daemon, Dis, would dominate the therapy and dictate her outer life. It was that possessed little girl within whose fears and beliefs dictated what was deemed safe, what feelings were safe, what people were safe, and how to control situations that felt unsafe. The kind of dissociation occurring within Eva is the severe form that happens early in a child's life, "well before the child's experience has been 'formulated' into complexes, and much more violent than repression" (Kalsched, 2023, p. 3). It appears to attack all connections between unwanted vulnerable parts of the self and the ego. What begins as an attempt to self-regulate becomes a mechanistic defense of the Self-care system (SCS), disconnecting feelings of pain and fear by controlling and dominating vulnerable parts of the self that seem to be the roots of pain and fear (Kalsched, 2023).

Integration of the Fragmented Self

One more dream emerged around this time that helped Eva and me more fully understand the enactments that occurred between us:

> *A toddler, familiar but not, no more than a year old, blond and white-faced, is spinning. He is spinning in a spaced-out way. I'm concerned he will get dizzy and throw up. He goes into my bathroom to throw up. There are two other young toddlers sitting inside the toilet, just quietly hanging out. I think the dream ends before he throws up, but I know that's the outcome because the other two toddlers become upset, realizing they are going to be thrown up on.*

As the dream ego, Eva's primary feelings were fear—that the boy might throw up—and upset, realizing that no one was aware of how gross it was for the kids to be in the toilet.

She goes on to say that she finds herself always looking for images of miserable children to use in her artwork. We explore how, from the time she was very young, she had to learn to dissociate her feelings and needs as a way to not further agitate her mother. Yet, at the same time, a part of her was "spun out" by her mom's anxiety, fear, and anger, and the family dynamics.

In the dream, a part of her can no longer hold in the nauseous agitation of being spun out—like me in the enactment. In the dream, the little ones in the toilet have learned to not know of their misery and don't want this state disrupted—like Eva in the enactment talking over me rather than tuning into herself as a way not to know, to keep fast to the dissociation. Now, together, we witness their misery. She and I, together, empathize with these very neglected parts of her that had to learn to accommodate the intolerable (Brandchaft, 1993). The dream helped her have enough distance to gain empathy. At this point in her analysis, if we were to talk directly about those parts of herself, she would not be able to take ownership or tolerate the associated affects. What becomes illuminated is that, as we empathize with these dream figures, Dis is not online/available to deny their existence or dismiss their needs and value.

The tensional field softens further as we make room for these realities. Eva reports how the dream makes her happy. Like her artwork, it depicts her experience and feelings accurately. Our growing ability to relate with each other about these feelings softens the accompanying shame. She more fully understands that the strategies and behaviors she had adopted were not because she was inherently "bad." Rather, they were the best way she could navigate an impossible and terrifying situation. Working with these insights and feelings helped her more fully integrate how difficult it was to sense her mother as a constant, reliable, and safe presence, and how this has played out with us. The enactments, as hard as they have been, are also illuminating. "[O]ne might say that the goal in working with enactments is to help the patient recognize the difference between feeling scared and feeling scarred" (Bromberg, 2011, p. 24).

Slowly, Eva was accepting the complexity of the dissociative processes, allowing for the inevitability of being thrown into the swirl of them again, yet experiencing that she could consciously track that process rather than be unconsciously spun out by it. As the shame softened, she could slow down inside and more fully accept the fragmentation she'd experienced, which paradoxically loosened its iron-clad grip.

In her early life, when her mother erupted and chased her, calling her stupid, the shock and accusations threw her into the grips of the Dark Angel (the negative pole of the SCS) and his unrelenting determination of her as "bad." And this would concretize in her as a shame-ridden identification. Being "good" was her only hope for survival, and this, too, would alternately concretize into a belief of what she absolutely had to be. And whichever pole she should find herself in, she would utterly adopt the inscribed identification and belief. Trapped in this situation, psychological integration of good and bad was not possible. Being held in the arms of the Bright Angel (the positive pole of the SCS) numbed the shock, fear, and protest that lived in her body.

A parentified child or "manager" would also readily take over when needed, in an attempt to control her mother (or me) when she had perceived her mother (or me) as incompetent. Meanwhile, in her outer life, the progressed adult could hold strong and function in a demanding job, and mother her daughters. These fragmented parts were the scars of trauma—they helped her survive but kept her from feeling.

In the early stages of the analysis, we worked to help Eva gain awareness of these distinctly different parts of herself by naming and giving them a voice. Her dreams would offer personifications, which helped her bring to life and differentiate what was muddled by the chaos within. We found a way for her to mock-up, in her body, the feel of the different parts and to have them dialogue with each other. She could tolerate only very short periods of this before a different part would intrusively jump in and hijack the show, cutting her off from feeling—often with a flood of words, associations, and information. In those times, I understood those shifts to be strategies to help her regulate, keeping her from too much feeling when we had overridden her window of tolerance.

In time, she internalized that focusing on her breath was the key to regulating the hypercharged states. We were then able to further this through something like interactive meditations. While integrating whatever feelings or images she brought into the session, we would do something like a guided meditation in which I would help her focus her awareness on her felt sensations specific to her experiences. With her breath serving as the candle in the dark, the light of consciousness was brought to sensations. Through our interactions, she could verbalize what her sensations felt like and what, if any, emotions, images, or memories arose. In this way, together, we worked to connect her psyche to her soma, slowly establishing a home within what Winnicott (1989/1964, p. 113) describes as psyche-indwelling soma.

The somatic work done within our relationship helped her bodily self to contain and ground the intense arousal that heretofore could not be borne, re-consolidating the relationship between her body and mind that had been disrupted so long ago. Re-finding and re-entering the tender heart of the very frightened little girl in this last session was deeply moving to both of us.

In Figure 7.3, Eva depicts an archetypal image of the Divine, Compassionate Feminine, holding in her gaze a woman whose relatives were in the holocaust. As the woman tells her story of grief and suffering from having relatives caught up in the holocaust, she brings her hand to her heart with compassion. This invokes Eva's courage to tell her story, including her grief and other feelings, with compassion for herself rather than shame and dismissal. Her immediate family was not directly involved in the holocaust, but they have relatives in Israel for whom the reality of the holocaust is very present. On the bottom left of the image are the bones of an infant found under an ancient road. There is new life, golden-colored, sprouting from this death. The image depicts the life–death–life cycle unfolding within her psyche.

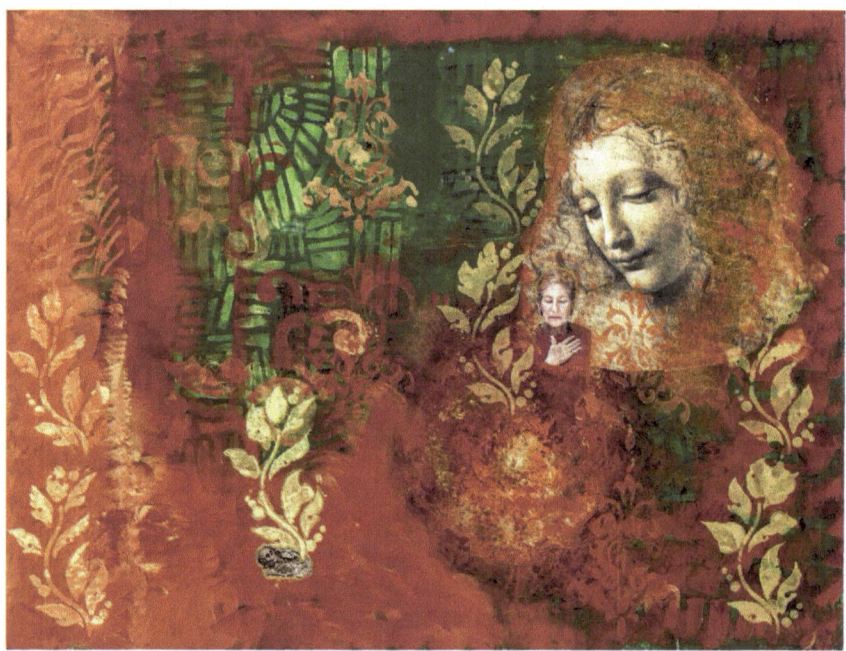

Figure 7.3 Compassionate, archetypal feminine gazes at grieving woman, new life emerging (Original artwork by Eva, with permission)

Eva's mother's primary trauma involved a sibling she was supposed to be watching over. The sibling was killed on the road in front of their house. Eva's mother felt responsible, though she was only a small child herself. The family could never verbally acknowledge to her that it was not her fault. Eva and I drew the link between the ancient road in her artwork and the road where her mother's sibling was killed. The transgenerational passage of trauma runs deep.

The Mythopoetic Gives Textured Meaning to Eva's Struggle Toward Embodiment

The Medusa Myth

Medusa first arose in Eva's collage painting. It was the snakes in Medusa's hair that gripped her attention. The image helped her remember that her mother had pulled Eva's hair out—events that were so painful and terrifying that she had dissociated the memory. And when she did remember, it was hard to hold onto it with much clarity. The first feeling that arose upon completion of the collage was that it was *accurate*—and thus deeply satisfying. It was later that Eva began to formulate that the Medusa and the bloody infant nursing at her breast symbolically represented her experience of her mother as dangerous, frightening, and attacking while simultaneously capturing that Eva had no choice but to seek nourishment from her regardless of this fact (see Figure 2.1). The image and feelings evoked were profoundly charged. The text she wrote on the back of the image read, "you are scaring and scarring me." In her analysis, creating conditions that allowed a co-regulation process was primary.

It wasn't until much later that the psychic space opened to explore her associations with the myth itself. She had not known the details of the myth. Bringing understanding to what shaped her mother's illness and behavior has been important in Eva's healing. Eva could hear that one of the central themes of the Medusa myth was at work in both her own and her mother's psyches—they both were denied a voice to their subjective experience, their own perspective, and feelings. She has come to understand the intrapsychic consequences of this.

The myth of Medusa has many versions. Medusa was a strikingly beautiful and sexual woman who had been raped by Poseidon in Athena's temple. Athena, unable to punish the powerful masculine god Poseidon, punished Medusa for desecrating her temple. She turned Medusa's golden hair into terrifying snakes. In this act, Medusa's pain was dismissed, and her rage boiled below, erupting in a gaze that turned to stone those who dared look at her. The hero Perseus cut Medusa's head from her body, which was applauded by the patriarchal powers. This act completely severed Medusa from her body, her source of feminine power and feeling. From a feminist perspective, Athena, distorted by her logos-dominated attitudes, betrays Medusa. "Medusa's beheading mythologizes the killing off of the wisdom aspects of the feminine, rooted in feelings in her body, and what remained is the one-sided representation of her destructive power" (Wirtz, 2021, p. 129). In the model of the Self-care system, the beheading is a depiction of the persecutory force that severs feelings in the body from consciousness. The traumatized psyche, petrified in a rigid and fragile structure, is not able to feel or contain affect and thus erupts when upset.

From the time she was very young, Eva was the recipient of that raw, uncontained, destructive power. In the early stage of our work, the negative aspect of the Self-care system was frequently symbolized in her dreams as a medieval knight wielding a sword in one hand and balancing in the other a tray on which stood a chalice full of wine. The sword, she came to understand, was aimed at cutting her head from her body, rendering her numb and feelingless. The wine depicted the near-addictive quality that drove the self-protective mechanisms aimed at keeping her from consciously feeling. It was a chaotic balancing act within. When she did indeed feel, the self-attack became ever more deriding or turned outward to attack me.

Artwork and Remembering in the Aftermath of Dissociation

Midway through her analysis, as her story began to take form, Eva brought in a doll she had made in an art group. It was of a young child with sores all over her head rather than hair. She began to remember how her mom would explode when Eva accidentally spilled something. Her mom would verbally attack, lunge for her hair, or chase Eva, and then ultimately pull her hair out. These events themselves were terribly traumatic, involving both physical attack and emotional abandonment. Eva's creative unconscious, over and over, has helped her remember what she had to dissociate to survive. It has served as a visual reminder that she and I returned to frequently, helping her to further formulate, clarify, symbolize, and integrate these episodic memories into long-term explicit memory.

Much of the somatically based work we have done is oriented toward regulating the intense states of hyper- and hypo-arousal associated with these events. The events stirred conflicting needs—to run/flee and, ultimately, dissociate/freeze from fear. The first stage of the traumatic experience was intense hyper-arousal, which was followed immediately by extreme life-threatening fear, leading to shutdown/dissociation/hypo-arousal. However, following such an event, Eva still needed to seek nourishment and proximity to her mom. She could only accomplish this by further splitting herself into parts while shutting down/dissociating her feelings of fear as well as any tender feelings that lay buried far below. The fluctuating and simultaneously occurring states of hyper- and hypo-arousal felt in relationship to her primary attachment figure created psychic disorganization and fragmentation. As is so when one has been severely traumatized, she has attempted to navigate these states through constant hyper-vigilance (Bromberg, 2011, p. 21).

Because the bond between her and her mother was disrupted so early, it upset the consolidation of her mind with her body and the achievement of "personalization" (Winnicott, 1965/1963, p. 223) or "indwelling of psych in the soma" (Winnicott,

1989/1964, p. 113). "When this optimal partnership does not occur, the baby prematurely turns away from the mother and toward the mind instead" (Winnicott 1949 in Kalsched, 2013, p. 286). Eva is very bright, accentuating her unconscious need for her mental capacity to "hold" her as her mother had not. Self-holding took the place of relying on another person. "The result is a defensive posture in which a 'pathological mind-psyche' (Winnicott, 1949, p. 244) is cathected by the infant in response to a failure of the holding environment" (Kalsched, 2013, p. 286).

The states of dysregulation were so highly charged and hard to navigate throughout her lifetime that shifting from feeling to thought became her default mode. Though understanding her dreams and piecing together an autobiographical narrative helped her gain a more coherent inner structure, moving into cognitive understanding always came with a risk of dissociation. Learning to let her feelings inhabit her body has shown to be her great alchemical work, where true transformation can happen. Based on this, it is only in the later stages of her analysis that we began to weave in the mythological ramifications of the Medusa story with hers. When we did, self-empathy took stronger root, and her perspective on her own experience widened, becoming less stigmatizing and shame-based.

In time, she linked the image of the Medusa to the attacking voice within her that shut down (turned to stone) any attempt toward conscious feeling or continuity of memory. In the final collage painting, reproduced in image 7.3, her feeling self, the soul–child within that seems to have died, is showing signs of new life which holds her potential—her potential to feel grief and tender feelings. As Jung says:

> One of the essential features of the child motif is its futurity. The child is the potential future … In the Individuation process, it anticipates the figure that comes from the synthesis of conscious and unconscious elements in the personality. It is therefore a symbol which unites the opposites; a mediator, bringer of healing, that is one who makes whole … I have called this wholeness that transcends consciousness the "self."
>
> (Jung, 1969/1954, p. 164)

Reclamation of an Embodied Self

Each stage of Eva's work could be viewed as titrating the layers of traumatic distress, orienting her on the long path of individuation. Throughout her analysis, her artwork seamlessly incorporated elements of her dreams and inner work. Through this, a mythopoetic narrative was woven that gave textured meaning to her struggle to feel her way into an embodied experience.

Jung reminds us again and again that psyche strives towards wholeness, toward psyche centered in Self rather than a splintered composite of parts. Yet, because this thrust toward wholeness can be disrupted by trauma, it is in a relationship with a responsive other, often a therapist, that it gets set back into motion. Once set in motion, "whether we consent or not … It is a mark of health to reach for madness in us" (Ulanov, 2020, p. 584). It is here that one can consciously suffer what occurred when one was too young to feel, understand, or integrate at the time or if, like Eva, one was so young that one's ego had not had time to organize into a cohesive sense of self. Winnicott's (1974) description of how it is that the worst has already happened, that the breakdown that is feared occurred in the past, can help us endure what inevitably must be relived in the analytic dyad, though this time in a homeopathic dose, so as not to retraumatize but to re-member and re-claim the split off pieces of the psyche—of the bodied-self.

The Case of Sally

The Star Draws Her to It: the Salt of Her Tears, the Depth of Her Body's Mystery and Beauty Found in Connection

Sally's deepest sense of meaning comes from knowing that she contributes, in the way that she can, to caring for our world and to our democracy. She is dedicated to consciously raising her three children. In the course of her analysis, she found meaningful work through building community and by accompanying others in the process of dying to facilitate their awakening to life. She learned to turn that same kind of caring and dedicated attention to herself that initially could only focus on the outer world. Early traumatic experiences had shattered a deeply personal knowing that she, too, mattered. In a letter to Ukrainian colleagues, Don Kalsched expressed the ineffable connection between democracy and consciousness:

> Your battle is part of that revolution in consciousness. Dictators will always rise up against this new consciousness because they are afraid of it, but the fight for democracy, for equality, for diversity, and for the sacred reality that all people on this planet contain the spark of a God-given right to life and liberty, is far bigger than any one battle, and it must be waged over and over again in every generation. Those of you who work with traumatized individuals know that this is the same battle waged in the inner world—between a life-promoting new, democratic consciousness and the violent, oppressive anti-life forces in the psyche … You are fighting for a new birth of freedom and for a new and revolutionary consciousness that is slowly taking place on this earth—against tremendous resistance. You are fighting for a transcendent moral center for your nation. Despite your current trauma, you are fighting for the Soul.
>
> (Kalsched, 2023, p. 1)

Sally suffered physical and emotional abuse at the hands of her father, who dominated the family in a dictatorial way. When she was 16, she was raped by a friend, throwing her into a state of shocked betrayal. Sally was 46 when we began working together. Though she had had a previous marriage and subsequent relationships, she was distressed that she had not formed the kind of intimate relationship with a man that she longed for. That vein of her psychic life had been insidiously hijacked by the negative Self-care system described by Kalsched, personified in Sally's dreams as a serial killer. She referred to him as a change agent. He had some uncanny prowess between the worlds of life and death. He would appear in her dreams each time change was brewing. Part of his prowess was that his behavior always seemed socially acceptable. This made him all the more menacing. In these dreams, she was the only one aware of his presence and intent. She threatened him because she could sabotage his desire to kill. However, she also felt powerless to stop him.

I was taken with her sense that she could sabotage his desire to kill. When I asked for more about this, she said she knew that if she called him out, she too could become his target, although she was unsure how she knew. In time, we both learned that to call him out meant to bring consciousness to his intent. Although this would be necessary to heal, it would also cause this archetypal protective force to double down on its intent to kill genuine feelings, her sense of aliveness. She told me this dream in the early phase of her analysis:

> *I'm at a conference for work. A man I have been attracted to and know to be a good father is doing the presentation. The conference hall is a steep theater with a stage at the bottom. The serial killer is there. Sometimes, he is walking about, so at times, I see him. He is aware that I'm aware of him. He has to find some socially acceptable way to kill me. He is looking for an opportunity. At times, he's in one of the conference hotel rooms, sometimes traveling through the hallways, and at times listening to the talk. I love the talk. Yet I am upset and distracted by my awareness of the killer.*

Sally, who is of European heritage, grew up in a working-class family in a multi-ethnic neighborhood of Chicago. She became the only child after her younger brother died when she was two. As time went on, the father, a former security officer, became more and more emotionally and physically abusive with both Sally and her mom. When Sally entered adolescence, he derided her body constantly. It seems he experienced Sally's aliveness as threatening. He ridiculed her accomplishments and dismissed the possibility that she was the author of her own works. When it was evident that Sally and a kind, caring young man had fallen in love, her father made certain that she did not have the freedom to leave the house to be with him. Each of these incidents, and many others that followed, could be likened to serial killings—attempts by her father's own defensive mechanisms to thwart Sally's life and inner spirit— because to allow for Sally's liveliness would require him to allow for his, which had begun to shut down long ago. His father, a former military officer, routinely used corporal punishment to teach his son to be a man. The death of his own son seemed to have sealed the deal—tender feelings were no longer bearable.

When Sally was 16, the father pinned her mother up against the wall by her throat, hit her, and kicked her. It took such an event, which Sally watched, for the mother to rise out of her distracted depression enough for her protective instincts to kick in. With a restraining order in place, the parents divorced.

In a session midway into our work, Sally tells me that when she was 10 years old, her father punched her so hard in the stomach that she blacked out. She began the following session by talking about Trump and his presidential campaign. We name, track, and titrate, via mindful awareness of her body-based experience, how being drawn into and unable to separate from the daily news about Trump is a reactivation of a state of vigilance that is all too familiar to her—paralleling what she had experienced as a child with her father. In time, we orient to how she is not now alone—unlike when she was growing up. In addition to me, many prominent women have validated her reality by publicly acknowledging that Trump's behavior of denigrating women is abusive.

From here, a deeper stratum of memory begins to arise. She speaks of a time when her Aunt Edith came to their house. Sally was a pre-teen. Hearing the father's abusive way with the family, Aunt Edith proclaimed that such abuse was not to be tolerated. And she left.

Sensing so much unmetabolized arousal as Sally speaks, I pursue it further, asking her to notice her inner experience as she remembers this. She lets me know that she experienced hope when her aunt, by naming her father's behavior as abusive, had validated her own experience. Yet, she still feels this anger toward her father simmering under the surface. Acknowledging her feelings, I ask her to notice what she is aware of in her body.

She gives something like a grimacing growl of exasperation, lifting her hand slightly—fingers gripped and shaking, saying, "I just want to rip his throat out."[7]

As I nod in recognition, she exhales strongly. I recognize a complete exhalation as an important cue that she is tolerating the sensations, thus allowing them to be felt and worked through rather than recirculating. By developing a capacity to feel, reflect on, and value her somatic experience, she can begin to inhabit the emergence of new possibilities more fully. I inquire about how it is inside now, and she responds, letting me know she feels relief and can breathe again.

We are quiet as that settles. Sally now remembers more—Aunt Edith didn't come back. Sally is now sitting in a very familiar posture, on the edge of the couch, crumped down over her stomach, looking like she is not breathing, yet making eye contact as she talks in an exasperated, resentful tone. When she sits this way, she seems to cut off from the possibility of sensing her body and, thus, from feeling. I also sense a grip in my stomach and am finding it hard to breathe. Based on all these perceptions, I pursue it further by asking, "As you remember that Aunt Edith didn't come back, what do you notice inside?" (Davies & Frawley 1994).[8]

She speaks of just feeling sluggish and crampy in her gut. I ask her to bring her awareness to her gut—we are quiet for a moment. Shrugging her shoulders, she says again, "Sluggish, it's just congested."

Embodied Sludge Resulting from Dis-missing Links between Body and Traumatic Memories

She is responding to the inquiry yet dismissing any meaningful link, instead verbally and nonverbally implying that she is too heavy, out of shape and hasn't been exercising enough, so that's just the way it is.

She seems to be letting me know that when she enters this inner territory, she meets such overwhelming *dis*couragement that she would rather not talk about it. The fact that we have just been discussing a memory seems to have disappeared. Shutting down she dissociates from her sensorial awareness and the memories that are rooted there—what Bion (1959) calls an attack on linking. This dissociative process hijacks her organism. There are no narrative memories here. In an attempt to make sense of what is going on inside, in comes what I referred to previously as a "story," of her being to blame for being sluggish and overweight, putting meaning to the implicit memory by Dis-ing herself and her body.

Empathizing with the distressing inner sensations and hoping she can attend to the felt/implicit memory without focusing on the content of ascribed meaning, I ask, "What is it like when you focus your awareness on the sensations in the congested place?"

She turns her attention inward. Because I know she can barely tolerate her inner experience and is apt to dissociate again by overriding the sensations and, instead, go to meaning, I do not let much time pass before I ask her what she notices.

She responds, letting me know that she feels a loosening. As tiny as this shift in her felt sense seems, from a somatic perspective, this is a necessary "titration"— that is, she is building tolerance, bit by bit, of the sensations that have been intolerable and dissociated heretofore.

I am aware my stomach is still quite gripped; I make use of my inner state to empathically inquire about hers by simply asking her what else she notices.

"Yeah, it is a little less tight." Then, "I don't know when Aunt Edith left … I felt hopeful but also dread. I knew she wouldn't come back. She'd be a target if she did."

I continue, "Hmm … like you were when he hit you in the stomach?" I link this to her having been his target, which she had spoken of in the previous session— connecting the affects of despair, dread, and terror to the memories, which had been held in her body but not linked to their root.

"Ugh—yeah," she exhales strongly as the recognition is felt square on.

There is a leaden pause—her eyes meet mine with feeling. Yet soon, Sally breaks in with: "Sometimes when we are doing this, I hear this resistance inside—like white noise."

Engaging the Felt Sensations of Shut Down: Encountering the Bright Angel of the Self-Care System

I ask her to say more about what that is like inside.

"Static, waves … like a pulsing wall."

I ask her, if the waves and static were in her body, where would they be?

She points to her chest and gestures with her hands, palms facing inward, making tiny quivering movements as they shake. I acknowledge her inner turmoil with my voice and nonverbal response. Now Sally brushes her hands across her chest like brushing stuff off and swiping it to the side. As she does this, I am aware I no longer feel engaged or moved as she gestures. I am not sure, but she seems to have overridden her direct experience and is gesturing to what she wishes would happen. I check out my perception by simply asking again what she notices inside.

She is still struggling; she has no words. The staticky feeling is still very present to me. I am unsure whether it is in her—like a state she cannot stay with—or between us, stemming from my pursuing the inquiry. It is a bit hard for me to think; I feel a sense of urgency and a loss of a basis of connection—perhaps this is what she is experiencing now but cannot put words to, and perhaps it is what she experienced at that time with her father.

From a somatically based trauma perspective, if a person is caught in a state of shutdown and is encountering an inner absence or a realm that has been dissociated, they may not be able to move through it by sensing the tensional field of the dissociated state itself. Being with the felt sense of an image of that experience, like the staticky, pulsing wall that Sally verbalized, will sometimes be enough to help a patient stay with and begin to tolerate the sensations so that something new can happen. However, if it does not facilitate a release from the shutdown state, an invitation to imagine and be with the felt sense of an opposite image can be useful. This can help the patient hold the tension of the opposites, which may simply not be available in that dissociated state. The transcendent function, somatically accessed, might thus activate. So, I ask her what an opposite image of the wall of static waves would be.

"A core thread of white light."

Again, when she speaks this, I notice I do not feel quite connected with her. Because of this, I suspect that though there is this image of a central inner core of light—which could organize the inner disorganization—I don't get a sense that she has actually experienced the felt sense of the image. It seems she would like to move on—but to do so would be to bypass the potential healing found in the image's felt experience. Or, it is possible that what she wants to move away from what she feels towards me? Based on the nature of the image—the bright light and her desire to move on—I am formulating that what might be afoot here is what Kalsched refers to as an abduction by the Bright Angel—the positive pole of the Self-care system. Making use of all of this, I ask her if she is okay to, again, carefully attend to her bodily-felt sensations.

She closes her eyes for a minute and sits much more upright. I see her breath moving through her torso, and she says, "More alert."

She does not elaborate; it is as if there is a blankness regarding how she could feel into this further and let it somatically move through. Though I can sense her attention pulling away and her desire to leave this dialogue, I know that if we move on without regulating the disrupted state, her nervous system's disorganizing arousal will not reorganize. Not surprisingly, there is an inner thrust to cognitively override her body experience and push on by finding meaning—a form of top-down coping. She dissociates while breaking the possibility of affective co-regulation between us (Schore, 2003). It seems likely that the disorganization and disruption between us is a re-living of the disorganized attachment pattern with her father. If she shuts down and moves away from intimacy, she doesn't feel it. But staying with what is happening between us revivifies it.

At the risk of being a bit dogged, but not wanting to be complicit with the dissociative process, I suggest simply staying with the experience, asking again what that is like inside, what the felt sense of alertness is like in her body.

She gestures down her torso and says, "Lighter. I feel more spacious ... yeah ... like safe."

This time, I can see that she has turned her attention inward, slowed down and thus has entered her felt sense more directly. She describes the sensations she is experiencing—and is allowing them to be felt bit by bit. As this happens, I feel the static and conflicting pulls I was aware of in me and between us begin to quiet. I see her bodily tension ease, and she settles. The feeling of connection between us is returning. Her breath is noticeably full; she is engaging me with eye contact. Her upper body is upright and her whole body is visibly engaged rather than being hinged forward at the hips, disconnecting her from feeling her lower body. Staying with her helped her find that she could be with the bodily-felt experience of this confusing inner territory. The two of us working together loosened the grip of the archetypal (non-human) Self-care system. A transformation that happens through human connection and affective co-regulation.

Pendulation, the Transcendent Function, and Developing Resiliency

Her tendency is to move immediately to meaning rather than further metabolizing this complex inner bodily state. I want to help her build on the felt experience in her body. By developing awareness, she can access and rely on it, building inner resilience, which increases her window of tolerance. I wonder aloud if she might invite that sluggish sensation to be present again, but this time right alongside the felt sense of the inner core of light. She focuses inward, and after a short bit, I see and hear a big exhale—which I take as a cue that the tensional field is reorganizing. She can again breathe and allow her vitality to return to this previously shutdown place.

Sally confirms this, saying, "The sluggish feeling dissipates even more. I feel lighter. Enlivened."

The archetypal force of the bright angel, which had been used in the service of defense, is humanized by our interaction. No longer polarized, it can now dwell with and transform the bodily-felt confusing static of dissociation. Our connection has been reinstated. The felt sense of the organizing image—a thread of white light inhabiting her core—soothes the panic that had manifested somatically as the staticky pulsing wall. I imagine this panic is what accompanied the original terror and immobilization. We have re-established a feeling of safety that was wholly disrupted when her father punched her. The implicit memory of this—the sense of not being safe and thus shutting down—arose between us when we got near the memory. Equal to the content of our interaction, Porges emphasizes,

> if you use prosodic intonation of voices—the tone is moving back and forth—it triggers in the nervous system a neuroception of safety, which detects those modulations as safety. The portal to change physiology can be through breath, but it also can be through listening … because as mammals our nervous system evolved the social engagement system (the myelinated vagal).
>
> (Porges, 2019, p. 20)

I ask her if it feels uncomfortable when I ask her to turn toward this part of herself.

"I want to change, not just talk forever; I want to, but at times I'm resistant."

I ask her if she has a sense of the resistance's function.

"It's the serial killer. He keeps things the same. Safe. He knows I see him—so like in dreams, he's trying to get me."

I respond empathically: "You survived by fighting. You came to know yourself as a fighter. However, your father hurt you. It must have been so terrifying. I wonder if the serial killer is trying to protect you from ever again feeling that vulnerable and scared?"

Sally's eyes fill with tears as she nods in affirmation. Before the session ends, we talk briefly about how hard it had been to be with this memory, but she now feels better from talking about it. We further explore how it seems that the serial killer aims to protect her by attempting to kill her consciousness of embodied feeling.[9]

In the next session, she recounts this dream:

> *There is an older woman from work, a matriarch. Being around her, I need to do these things—she places a requirement on my behavior.*

(Hearing this, I wonder whether I was too directive in the last session, and she accommodated my interventions.)

> *She is a role model—ambassadorial, supportive. I want to be there when she is there. She gets what I am working on and supports me in taking it to a higher level. She is validating. She encourages me to rise up. She can be vulnerable. Admits mistakes, which I don't easily. She is a counterpoint to the serial killer, who is like a wall that I bump into. I want to hit him (it) and say, "Fuck you." But it is safer to please him, stay where I am, and put a lid on myself.*

The meaning she draws from the dream counters my concerns about being overly directive. She tells me of someone she is newly dating—the first time in a year and a half. He is excited about her, and she about him. She says she feels she has grown in herself.

A Resurgence of Dis: the Serial Killer Returns

Though I did not expect it then, in retrospect, it is understandable that Sally risking vulnerable feelings in this new relationship and with me would be followed by a major resurgence of the serial killer. The inner defensive mechanisms, personified archetypally as Dis and internalized in Sally's psyche as a serial killer, do not give up easily.

Her next dream:

There is a really, really muscular, testosterone-y monster. I was doing battle with him. I had a blade. I sliced his chest. It bled gold—chelated this gold substance that would make it heal. Others, silent and behind me, were there fighting him, too. He would be cut, but he was healing because of the gold, and the gold was making him more beautiful. I was intrigued by the gold chelate and his reaction. We were getting a lot of blows in, and we intended to harm him. But it seemed to make him triumphant ... At times, I clawed his chest and ripped it—the gold came out—he laughed. There was no wounding him or taking him down. I was perplexed but didn't feel I was losing. I felt clarified. He needed to know I would fight back—this fantastical monster— I'm showing you my power. I am coming after you, motherfucker. I am not running.

I woke and felt it was the new incarnation of the serial killer but creepier— like he can fly under the radar.

Without missing a beat, she tells me how now, when she is at her father's house, if he becomes abusive to his wife, she chastises him, saying, "I don't ever want you to say that in my presence." She further says, "He listens now; it changes the energy."

Through our relating to this persecutorial archetype as it has lived in her, she is beginning to relate to it, both within and with others, thus humanizing it. In so doing, she develops agency and choice instead of letting it run her behavior unbidden.

Continuing in an upsurge of memory, she speaks of how, while growing up in such a rough neighborhood of Chicago, she always had to figure out who was dangerous and who was not. It seemed that men dominated family and cultural life. She tells me how, as a teen, one of her peers protected her and later wanted her to marry him. She says that all his life, his father beat him. Now, he lives in a trailer and is a butcher. She adds, "He's probably a serial killer."

She wonders whether the man she is dating will be protective. Then comes an inner onslaught of the serial killer—she says to herself—"My stomach is gross! He's not attracted to me!" But soon, she buffers it with a tone that conveys, "Oh yeah, here it is." But that experience is now outdated; she understands her old attempt to be perfect, not to feel vulnerable.

Sally once told me that when her father hit her, it was like a drug. She would want to fight him, take him on. The adrenaline release of the sympathetic fight/flight arousal never resolved. Thus primed and repetitively reactivated, the adrenaline rush became addictive. This repetitive impulse to fight had become entrapping, keeping her from loving. Her work now is to turn this aggression in service of the ego—to fight for what she loves and values.

A Redemptive Dream: from Dis-aster to Reconnecting with Her Star's Inner Guidance

In the following session, she shares this dream:

> I'm on a moonscape kind of beach—reddish dirt—like the Great Salt Lake. I think of it like a city beach in San Francisco—it has the potential to be beautiful, but there is such a human impact. A friend, Ellie, is with me and says, "I have something to show you." We climb up this crest and see the beautiful blue lake with a star over it. Ellie says, "See? This is the beauty of the world." What a treasure. I am thinking of how much I love her and will miss her—she's leaving the company. She is a manager who has not been recognized for her work and is no longer willing to stand for that. What a treasure she is. She took my arm from behind and we are smiling at each other looking out over the lake. It was twilight; the sky was a deep blue, like just after sunset.

Sally and I are both moved by the beauty of the dream and enter into a tender tone of connection simply through her telling of it. Much of the dream's significance feels like the experience of the dream itself. I gently ask her where she experiences it in her body.

She says her heart and how her arms, hands, and legs are tingling. We linger there in the nonverbal—the quivering numinosity of beauty and the feeling of our connection deepening.

Her associations follow later: "We appreciate each other," she says. "It's like a female equivalent to a romance. We felt wonder and joy at the crest. In the hard scrabble of the world, there is this untrodden beauty that humans can't touch."

Sally says spontaneously, "I am going to miss you, Ellie ... but I know you will be around."

She then says, "It's about change. I have a big feeling things are going to be okay—a feeling of the reassurance of closeness and persistent immutable friendship."

Her dream eloquently expresses the tender experience of feeling that our connection is reliable and that this is possible with others, too. Secure attachment is the lived experience of activating the vagal nerve that mediates social engagement. Her psyche reassuringly expresses that, although the wounding she has suffered has impacted her a great deal, within her is a divine innocence that has not been destroyed.

Regarding the star, she says, "It is something to guide us and to focus on. The salt is like my tears."

I ask about the inland lake.

"Like my body ... you don't know what's in the depths of it. The star draws you to it and lets you know something—but it is deep, mysterious. A new leaf, the dream is redemptive."

I say, "You have been through so much in your body."

Sally says, "So many women I know have. So has everyone."

I ask, "Is that how the serial killer goes about his work but in a socially acceptable way? Though what you just said may be quite true in our culture and worthy of acknowledgment, does that move of generalizing, and thus minimizing what you have experienced, take you away from the tender, vulnerable feelings you were just with?"

She visibly settles back into herself, opens again to the feeling of our connection, and nods to me in recognition. There is a softening.

The session ends. I wonder whether I was killing the moment with unnecessary empathy and then an interpretive response that took her out of her window of tolerance for tender feelings.

Disaster, an operation of Dis, means to become separated from your stars (Kalsched, 2013). Sally's experience of trauma resulted in the loss of her guiding star— her ability to trust in her own beauty and capacity to love and be loved.

Although I had wondered whether my intervention at the close of our last session had been too harsh, Sally opened the next session with no sign of empathic break: "I want to let go of my abusive father. Pull up the root and dead plant of it—of not having a father I can trust. I am worthy of being loved and treated tenderly. Anger just feeds on itself. Underneath it is grief and loss."

Embodied Active Imagination

I ask her what part of her feels that loss and grief. She tells me the young one, the 10-year-old. From here, we worked with an active imagination that emphasizes staying with the felt sense in her body. I ask what she would say if she were to gesture to that young one. She closes her eyes and tells me she would just pick her up and hold her in her lap. I ask if she can imagine being the 10-year-old in Sally's lap. "What is it like in your body to feel held by Sally?" Quietly, she indicates that, in her chest and belly, there is a feeling of warmth, love, and safety. I encourage her to give herself time with that.

After a bit, I ask her whether she can now feel what it feels like to be the adult holding the little one. With an affirming nod, she shifts to the perspective of the adult. I wonder how it feels in her body to be the one holding this little one. She describes how she feels the little one's warm weight and loves how she leans into her chest. She stays with the felt sense, acknowledging via the prosody of her voice the tenderness of feeling, allowing her body to let her know what it is that she needs. She is now the holder and the held.

Full Circle: Deepening Embodied Meaning

In the following session, she tells me about the tender lovemaking with her boyfriend and how good she feels: open, loved, vulnerable, and how she is feeling much more loving to herself.

In a later session, she reveals how, over a year ago, she had panicked and fled when the possibility of a feeling-full encounter had arisen with a man she admired. At the time, she had internally attacked herself, saying, "What's wrong with me?" This encounter had been with the man who gave the talk in the initial dream recounted in this section. Now, she and I were able to link that state of panic and need to flee with the feeling that arose for her when working with the memory of having been punched in the stomach by her father. Panic and the need to flee were also associated with the trauma incurred when she was raped at 16. We worked with this at a later time, linking the same dynamic—panic and the need to flee that had been stifled at the time of the trauma. When the panic arose in the past, it left her very confused about getting close to a man. Together, we could empathize with the panicky confusion and why it had activated with the possibility of opening to what she most longs for.

Initially, Sally referred to the serial killer as a change agent. However, she came to recognize that although he appeared each time change was brewing, he was actually an anti-change agent. Throughout this phase of her analysis, she painstakingly worked through traumatic memories, which allowed her to indwell her body more fully. Not only could she be with her genuine feelings, but she also began to bring her tender feelings into a relationship with another.

In *The Vision Seminars*, Jung states:

> You see, if your soul is detachable as in the primitive condition, you are simply hypnotized into a sort of somnambulist state or a trance, and whatever you experience in that condition is not felt because it has not been experienced in the body; you were not there when it happened. Only if you first return to the body, to your earth, can individuation take place, only then does the thing become true.
>
> (Jung, 1997, p. 1314)

Rather than the notion that primitive peoples inhabit primitive states, I believe such primitive states occur in all of us when our organism is highjacked by evolutionarily primitive parts of our nervous system. When a perceived threat hijacks our nervous system, it throws us into fight, flight, or dissociation. For those of us who have experienced that level of trauma, as well as for the clinician working with these states, we know just how vexing the way back into the body can be. Indigenous cultures often refer to the healing of such states as soul retrieval, requiring the presence of a medicine person. Jungian analysts have traditionally looked to the dream.

However,

To experience a dream and its interpretation is very different from having a tepid rehash set before you on paper. Everything about this psychology, is in the deepest sense, experience; the entire theory, even where it puts on the most abstract airs, is the direct outcome of something experienced.

(Jung, 1966/1943, p. 199)

The growing body of psycho-physically based trauma studies and neuroscience confirms how essential it is to attend to the complex unfolding of the somatic experience in the healing of trauma. It is when the psyche indwells the soma that we can begin to experience a sense of our full personhood and the numinous recognition of a vital spark at the center of our being—a sense of being on this earth, aligned with our star (Winnicott, 1960).

Notes

1 See Don Kalsched's 2023 article on Inner and Outer Democracy: With the Ukrainian Jungians in Webinar #8, Archive for Research in Archetypal Symbolism, webinars from the #WithUkranianJungians project. https://aras.org/wujwebinars

2 Additional sources for the work of Somatic Experiencing include P. A. Levine (1997, 2015). Training can also be found on the websites of Somatic Experiencing International and Ergos Institute.

3 The psychological "transcendent function arises from the union of conscious and unconscious contents" (Jung 1960, p. 69). When the conscious attitude becomes too one-sided, the unconscious behaves in a complimentary or compensatory manner—and vice versa.

4 Thích Nhất Hạnh (1926–2022) was a Vietnamese Thiền Buddhist monk and peace activist recognized as the inspiration for engaged Buddhism. He holds an important place in Eva's psyche.

5 Historians have found references to qigong-like techniques from at least 5,000 years ago. The practice emerged in China as people observed ways in which life was nurtured in plants and animals, and then were moved to embody these principles. See *History of Qigong* (2018) by Lee Holden and LeAnn Meyer. www.holdenqigong.com/history-of-qigong/, June 5, 2018. Retrieved October 30, 2023.

6 See Davies and Frawley (1994, pp. 168–171) regarding the unseeing and uninvolved parent and the neglected child, and the revivification of these dynamics in the transference/countertransference. Eva and I were able to turn to these dynamics at another time.

7 See Wirtz (2021/2014, p. 124): "Feeling and expressing the rage and chaotic despair in a contained manner can be a way of reclaiming the body, of redeeming the part of the self that got crushed in the violent experience. Cultural imprinting usually does not allow women to act out their aggressiveness and their fantasies of power. Consequently, the repressed rage is turned inward into severely self-harming behaviors that stifle and deplete their energy."

8 See Davies and Frawley (1994) on the significance of an abused child having a sense that someone sees and protects them from abuse, or the dynamics that arise when there is an absence of a sense of a witness or protector. If I had not continued to acknowledge what occurred when Aunt Edith left, I would also have become one who saw but did not protect.

9 Kalsched (2023, p. 3) emphasizes that the negative aspect of the SCS "operates to kill our awareness of pain that has been unbearable or to anesthetize our painful feelings in general, so they never become conscious. And it leads inevitably to [an inner and outer] authoritarianism." Comment in square parentheses added.

References

Bion, W. R. (1959). *Attacks on linking, second thoughts* (pp. 86–92). New York: Jason Aronson.

Brandchaft, B. (1993). To free the spirit from its cell. In A. Goldberg (Ed.), *The widening scope of self psychology* (pp. 209–230). Hillsdale, NJ: Analytic Press. https://doi.org/10.4324/9780203778951

Bromberg, P. M. (2011). *The shadow of the tsunami and the growth of the relational mind.* New York: Routledge.

Chodorow, J. (1999/1978). Dance therapy and the transcendent function. In P. Pallaro (Ed.), *Authentic movement: Essays by Mary Starks Whitehouse, Janet Adler, and Joan Chodorow* (p. 247). London: Jessica Kingsley.

Cwik, A. J. (2011). Associative dreaming: Reverie and active imagination. *Journal of Analytical Psychology, 56*(1). https://doi.org/10.1111/j.1468-5922.2010.01888.x

Davies, J. M., & Frawley, M. G. (1994). *Treating the adult survivor of childhood sexual abuse: A psychoanalytic perspective.* New York: Basic Books.

Grotstein, J. (2000). *Who is the dreamer who dreams the dream: A study of psychic presences.* Hillsdale, NJ: Analytic Press.

Herbert, B. M., Herbert, C., & Pollatos, O. (2011). On the relationship between interoceptive awareness and alexithymia: Is interoceptive awareness related to emotional awareness? *Journal of Personality, 79*, 1149–1175.

Holden, L., & Meyer, L. (2018). *History of Qigong.* www.holdenqigong.com/history-of-qigong/, June 5, 2018. Retrieved October 30, 2023.

Jung, C. G. (1960). The transcendent function. In *The structure and dynamics of the psyche. Collected works, vol. 8.* London: Routledge & Kegan Paul.

——— (1963). *Mysterium coniunctionis.* R. F. C. Hull (Trans.). *Collected works, vol. 14.* New York: Bollingen Foundation.

——— (1966/1943). On the psychology of the unconscious. In *Two essays on analytic psychology. vol. 7, collected works.* Princeton, NJ: Princeton University Press.

——— (1969/1954). *The archetypes and the collective unconscious.* R. F. C. Hull (Trans.), *vol. 9, collected works.* Princeton, NJ: Princeton University Press.

——— (1997). *Visions: Notes of the seminar given in 1930–1934.* C. Douglas (Ed.). Princeton, NJ: Princeton University Press.

Kalsched, D. (1996). *The inner world of trauma: Archetypal defenses of the personal spirit.* London: Routledge.

———— (2013). *Trauma and the soul: A psycho-spiritual approach to human development and its interruption.* New York: Routledge.

———— (2020). Opening the closed heart: Affect-focused clinical work with the victims of early trauma. *Journal of Analytic Psychology, 65*(1), 136–152.

———— (2023). Inner and outer democracy and the threat of authoritarianism: "With Ukrainian Jungians," from the text of Webinar # 8, September 19, 2023, Archive for Research in Archetypal Symbolism, webinars from the #WithUkranianJungians project. https://aras.org/wujwebinars

Levine, P. A. (1997). *Waking the tiger.* Berkeley: North Atlantic Books.

———— (2010). *In an unspoken voice: How the body releases trauma and restores goodness.* Berkeley: North Atlantic Books.

Levine, P. A. (2015). *Trauma and memory: Brain and body in a search for the living past: A practical guide for understanding and working with traumatic memory.* Berkeley: North Atlantic Books.

Lynd, H. M. (1958). *On shame and the search for identity.* New York: Harcourt Brace.

Modell, A. H. (1993). *The private self.* Cambridge, MA: Harvard University Press.

Muller, L. E., Shultz, A., Anderman, M., Gabel. A., Gesher, D. M., Spohn, A., Herpertz, S. C. & Bertsch, K. (2015). Cortical representations of afferent bodily signals in borderline personality disorder: Neural correlates and relationship to emotional dysregulation. *JAMA Psychiatry, 72*, 1077–1086.

Paulus, M. P., & Stein, M. B. (2010). Interoception in anxiety and depression. Brain Structure and Function, 214(5–6), 451–463.

Porges, S. (2001). The polyvagal theory: Phylogenetic substrates of a social nervous system. *International Journal of Psychophysiology, 42*(2), 123–146.

———— (2009). The polyvagal theory: New insights into adaptive reactions of the autonomic nervous system. *Cleveland Clinic Journal of Medicine, 76*(4–2), S86–S90. www.ncbi.nlm.nih.gov/pmc/articles/PMC3108032/

———— (2019). Rethinking trauma: Polyvagal theory can revolutionize your work with trauma survivors. An interview with Ruth Bucznski at the National Institute for the Clinical Application of Behavioral Medicine. https://s3.amazonaws.com/nicabm-stealthseminar/Rethinking-trauma-new/Stephen/NICABM-StephenPorges_Part5-Transcript.pdf

Ringstrom, P. (2007). Scenes That write themselves: Improvisational moments in relational psychoanalysis. *Psychoanalytic Dialogues, 17*(1), 69–99. https://doi.org/10.1080/1048 1880701301303

Russell, P. (1999). Trauma and the cognitive function of affects. In J. G. Teicholz, & D. Kriegman (Eds.), *Trauma, repetition, & affect regulation: The work of Paul Russell.* London: Rebus Press.

Schore, A. N. (2003). *Affect regulation and repair of the self.* New York: W. W. Norton.

Segal, H. (1973). *Introduction to the Work of Melanie Klein.* London: Routledge.

Stein, M. (1998). *Jung's Map of the Soul.* Peru, IL: Open Court Publishing.

Ulanov, A. (2020). The agony of integration and the blessings of finitude: Facing "extinction points" and moments of madness. *Journal of Analytic Psychology, 65*(3), 584–599. https://doi.org/10.1111/1468-5922.12601

Whitehouse, M. (2007). Physical movement and personality. In P. Pallaro (Ed.), *Authentic movement: Essays by Mary Starks Whitehouse, Janet Adler and Joan Chodorow.* London: Jessica Kingsley.

Winnicott, D. W. (1949). Mind and its relation to the psyche-soma. In *Through pediatrics to psycho-analysis.* (pp. 243–254). New York: Basic Books.

———— (1960). The theory of the parent–infant relationship. *International Journal of Psycho-Analysis*, *41*, 585–595.

———— (1965/1963). The mentally ill in your caseload. In *The maturational process, and the facilitating environment*. New York: International University Press.

———— (1989/1964). Psycho-somatic illness in its positive and negative aspects. In C. Winnicott, R. Shepherd, & M. Davies (Eds.), *Psycho-analytic explorations* (pp. 482–492). Cambridge, MA: Harvard University Press.

———— (1974). Fear of breakdown. International Review of Psycho-Analysis, 1(1–2), 103–107.

Wirtz, U. (2021). *Trauma and beyond: The mystery of transformation*. London, New York: Routledge.

Chapter 8

The Body as Experienced by the Therapist

Throughout history, healers, medicine people, and therapists have tried to compre-hend the complex and sometimes chaotic nature of their experience with those they treat. This can be traced back to ancient times, when medicine people explored the vast array of psychophysical–spiritual realms that often manifest during the intense and highly activated interactional field that unfolds between themselves and those seeking help. These healers described being psychically infected by or taking on the illness of the patient. Psychophysical dismemberment and near-death experi-ences demanded a personal journey on the part of the healer (psychic, spiritual, and bodied) to restore health and balance within themselves while simultaneously restoring health in the one seeking treatment. Not infrequently, these journeys were understood as initiatory, which, if survived, instilled inner strength and wisdom, en-hancing the consciousness of the healer (Eliade, 1964; Halifax, 1990). The healer–initiate's transformation was often perceived as a journey through multiple realms of reality, including elemental, plant, animal, and imaginary and territorial realms such as underwater, underground, earthly, bodily, psychic, and cosmic. A medicine person's experience of death and rebirth constellated numinous energies that aided both healer and patient through illness and to renewal.

These stories have fascinated many psychotherapists, including myself, because the accounts describe something of what we encounter working with others (van Löben Sels, 2019; Sedgewick, 1994). Jung (1966/1946) understood these histor-ical accounts within the mythical context of the wounded healer. The wounded healer has gained personal knowledge of disease through the direct experience of suffering. On the positive pole of the archetype, the wounded healer has suffered dis-ease consciously and thus can accompany another through conscious suffer-ing. The negative pole is represented by one who, having not suffered consciously remains prone to unconscious projection, the impulse to fix or give advice, affec-tive reactivity, and other forms of acting out that hamper an ability to be present for and with another's suffering. The dramatic descriptions imagistically express what therapists, healers, and patients sometimes *feel* unfolding within. They also dramatically portray reciprocal entwinement.

Psychoanalytic thinkers have come a long way in conceptualizing what hap-pens within. The bedrock of psychoanalytic understanding is based on Freud's

DOI: 10.4324/9781003305804-9

recognition of the unconscious, including transference and countertransference dynamics, and Jung's addition of the collective unconscious. Today, dismemberment and rebirth, while still containing a somatic dimension, might symbolize dissociation and re-memberment.

In *The Psychology of the Transference* (1966/1946), Jung articulated the vectors of communication that analyst and analysand inevitably enter in their encounter: conscious to conscious, unconscious to unconscious, conscious to unconscious, and unconscious to conscious. Through containment, reflection, and attention to the arising of their own unconscious and preconscious material, the analyst processes these communications and brings them into the dialogue with the patient, furthering the treatment. Jung recognized the degree to which both members of the dyad were affected by the other, and that, for an analysis to be effective, both would necessarily be transformed. He began to depict how the analyst could suffer a psychic infection of his patient's illness—as unconscious psychological dis-ease was transferred from patient to doctor.

In this context, Jung recognized the somatic unconscious and how the analyst may experience psychophysical disturbances resulting from interactions with the patient. "It is inevitable," Jung writes,

> that the doctor should be influenced to a certain extent, and even that his nervous health should suffer. He quite literally "takes over" the sufferings of his patients and shares them with him. For this reason, he runs a risk and must run in the nature of things.
>
> (1966/1946, para 358)

While Jung recognized this mutual influence and the body as a part of that, he did not allude to the fuller notion of embodiment. More recently, interaffectivity—coordinated interaction, bodily resonance, and mutual incorporation—has been used to describe the embodied, circular affective interaction between individuals that provides the basis for primary empathy and how, through their interactions, two individuals become a part of each other's lived experience (Fuchs, 2017) whether or not unconscious processes primarily drive the interaction.

Mirror Neurons, Projective Identification, and Enactments

For decades, psychoanalysts have used Melanie Klein's concept of projective identification (1952) to understand the otherwise often inexplicable levels of involvement induced within the analytic dyad. Sedgewick (2014) historically traces how Klein's ideas on projective identification arose in the same year Jung wrote,

> The doctor, by voluntarily and consciously taking over the psychic sufferings of the patient, exposes himself to the overpowering contents of the unconscious and hence also to their inductive action .... The patient, by bringing an activated

unconscious content to bear upon the doctor, constellates the corresponding unconscious material in him.

(1966/1946, p. 176)

Unlike Klein, Jung did not view such communications on the part of the patient as aggressive or defensive. Instead, he perceived it to be a matter of course, saying, "Doctor and patient thus find themselves in a relationship founded on mutual unconsciousness" (1966/1946, p. 176). Sedgewick reflects on how such a situation is ripe for enactments.

More recently, Bromberg (2011) and other relational analysts have shown how this is so by depicting enactments as a scenario in which the unexpected loss of relational coherence drives the analytic encounter into chaotic disarray. If the therapist navigates these chaotic states in collaboration with the patient, they potentially make way for a new relational organization to emerge. Jung's 1935 comment, "No longer is he [the analyst] the superior wise man, judge, and counselor; he is a fellow participant who finds himself involved in the dialectical process just as deeply as the so-called patient" (1966/1935, p. 8), deeply resonates with my experience of the enactments described in Chapter 7 with my patient, Eva. I was humbled by the forces at work as I soon understood that an intelligence had arisen between us and guided us into territory neither could access through our conscious volitions. Perhaps based on the newly balanced symmetry between us, Eva could be with what had been inaccessible heretofore—the melting of a bodily-based self-protective dissociative freeze about her heart—a re-membering of feeling the possibility to feel that had been dissociated. In the fresh ground of our shared vulnerability (BC-SPG, 2013), there arose an expanded capacity to be with and reflect on both of our behaviors, allowing her to navigate the affective territory of her core wound.

The body is rarely, if ever, included in descriptions of projective identification or enactments. The discovery of mirror neurons has illuminated the centrality of the body in both. In the analytic encounter, we are not somatically detached from the interaction. Via mirror neurons, our bodies resonate with the actions of the other. We sense the patient's affective expression and potential meaning through our mirror neuron's prospective function and, in response, our body prepares itself to interact (Ammaniti & Ferrari, 2013). The patient's body communicates explicit and implicit patterns of relational organization through facial expressions, muscular patterns of relational conflict, dynamics, subtle gestures, or the absence of gestures and intonations of voice, though these can be nearly imperceptible to an observer.

The communications are mediated through mechanisms that include the mirror neuron system, adaptive oscillators, and other yet-to-be-known mechanisms that induce somatic synchrony and imitation in the observer–therapist (Stern, 2018/1985). The mirror neuron system is stimulated not only to imitate but to predict the intent and meaning of a patient's bodily movements *which are an intrinsic aspect of* emotional expressions. When movement and emotional expressions are observed rather than imitated, the actual motoric execution is inhibited even though the motor network is activated (Gallese, 2009, pp. 522–523).

Thus therapists, in their containing function, simulate in their own bodies the patient's movement and emotional expression, but they do not take it into action. Nearly simultaneously, the therapist simulates their own bodily-based response to the patient. Unless the therapist is purposefully tracking their own somatic experience, such processes typically unfold outside of awareness. However, whether consciously aware or not of their inner somatic realm, the therapist's psyche-soma registers the information. "The notion of projective identification and the interpersonal dynamic related to transference and countertransference can be viewed as instantiations of the implicit and prelinguistic mechanisms of the embodied simulation-driven mirroring mechanisms" (Gallese, 2009, p. 531).

A multitude of conflictual scenarios the therapist may be containing can be imagined. For example, if the patient is feeling destructive aggressive impulses—these forces are activated and simulated in the therapist's body. If the therapist's organic response would be to move away from someone threatening violence, and yet the therapist has a history of being trapped rather than free to move, that action–tension is also simulated in their body (Gallese, 2012, Gallese & Guerra, 2019). Now, the therapist is containing these conflictual action patterns. While the therapist's self-reflective function can metabolize conflictual affects and impulses, they can also be overwhelmed and unable to do so adequately until the session ends and there is enough psychic space for reflection and somatic unwinding. If one or more sessions immediately follow in which the therapist is yet again left, literally somatically holding traumatically based unprocessed scenarios, it is not surprising that they might find their psyche soma depleted and taxed.

While we can now more fully understand ourselves as interactants in the interaffective field rather than passive recipients of the patient's unconscious communication, our nervous systems nonetheless can and do sometimes feel captured by the patient. In that interaction, though the therapist's core sense of self is not entirely coopted, there is a degree of organistic matching (mirrored simulation) of the patient's impulses and self-protective mechanisms. These may be subdued or amplified in the therapist through collision or in collusion with the therapist's own inner self-protective mechanisms and tendencies, whether conscious or unconscious. Additionally, when the therapist knows firsthand something of the affective challenge the patient struggles with (not specific content but depth of affective quality and process), a powerful embodied resonance is set in motion for both (Fuchs & Koch, 2014).

Purposeful awareness brought to bear on the unfolding somatic processes potentiates a deeper capacity for felt attunement, empathy, and the emergent embodied meaning arising between the two. I have defined attunement and empathy as I use and understand these terms in Chapter 4. Having empathy for a patient allows the analyst to further inquire, from a place of understanding how or why it is a patient may feel or act a certain way. Inquiry from that place does not solely mean emotional alignment with the patient's position but being in a related place from which one can inquire while respecting the patient's subjective experience. It may lead to analytic engagement/confrontation—but confrontation by feeling and understanding the patient's adaptive choices rather than potentially shaming or judging.

Such engagement, without empathic understanding is likely to not only induce shame but also increase the likelihood of bogging down in resistance or conflict. Analytic engagement, of course, includes responses that effectively move the dyad toward connection or needed distancing and boundaried reactions.

To the degree that the patient or therapist's own affective experience is unformulated or not fully processed, the therapist's inner capacity to stay the course over time is the light guiding both of them through the unformulated, murky darkness of the underworld (Cwik, 2011). The reality of the body and mirror neuron system does not do away with projective identification, whether felt, imagined, or theoretically conceived. Perhaps most importantly, it adds another felt dimension, which can enhance the therapist's reverie as it opens and receives the analysand's psychic process. In this holding environment, the analyst's and analysand's dreams and other expressions of the creative unconscious, including somatic experience, relational processing, and insights, also, of course, move the work along. Because there is always more that can be brought to one's consciousness, the therapist will always be affected to some degree as they accompany those with whom they work.

In the therapist's use of self, their own bodily sensations, energetic waves of sensations, postures, tensional dynamics in the deep body and viscera, slight movements, and gestures can offer meaningful information, feeling, and insight into what is going on in themselves, in the analysand and between the two. For some, like myself, matching, resonating, mirroring, or otherwise sensing my patient's bodily states often cues me into levels of anxiety, aversion, contempt, fear, anger, rage, and dissociative processes unfolding long before they are revealed verbally by the patient. (It is important to note that what I or another therapist might experience in that process is likely to be only a tiny percent of the activation the patient experiences.) Further empathic inquiry with the patient can confirm or deny the accuracy of one's understanding of those bodily cues—with simple questions like, "I wonder what you notice you are experiencing inside? Or I wonder if you are feeling contempt right now?" All of which can be extremely helpful—correcting, confirming, or opening a path of analytic engagement.

The existence of mirror neurons and other biologically based ways in which we are cued into the other's behavioral and emotional intent also does not imply absolute emotional empathic knowing of the other. In addition to verbal exploration with the analysand, the therapist's continual self-reflection as to what it stirs in themselves is ever needed. These reflections need to be sorted through for a useful therapeutic response to be offered.

When analytic listening is extended to include the somatic dimension, the therapist might experience in their own body what has been implicitly known or pre-reflectively experienced by the patient—especially preverbal and traumatic experience. Taking Jung's measured statement, "It is inevitable, that the doctor should be influenced to a certain extent, and even that his nervous health should suffer" (1966/1946, para. 358) into the consulting room has a different feel than it reads. Because we are much more than a nervous system, the actual lived experience of being the therapist in such a situation is *fleshed out*. In Chapter 4, I further described how I was influenced in the course of my work with Lucinda. In that phase of our work, Lucinda found herself repetitively caught up in a particular affective dilemma that played out in several relationships. The unformulated quality of the affect was underscored through the repetition and her difficulty dropping down into genuine feeling. I was troubled by the impasse. I felt immersed in an atmospheric, murky quality of affect that made it hard for me to find a way to productively engage. A layer of my own implicit memory had been activated. I became aware of this when a dream woke me with an embodied memory of terror distinctly present in my body. Though the memories and affects were painful, a newfound clarity was born in me from attending to them. I had often addressed that phase of my life in my own analysis, but attending anew to what had been activated between us deepened my capacity to meet her in an attuned, empathic way.

Engaging Lucinda in that highly activated psychophysical field was not simple. What was crucial was to directly contact her memories and feelings while carefully safeguarding her from being flooded by sensations, emotions, and memories that would only retraumatize her. While the methods of SE were incredibly useful, being open to knowing more of my own inner territory was essential. It allowed me to be grounded and see it through, eventually bringing the feelings induced in her early wound to bear in the here and now between us. My own inner work opened a passageway for her to enter the difficult territory she needed to address. Reciprocally, Lucinda's work furthered mine.

Discreet self-disclosure of the therapist's own somatic phenomena can be as useful as the therapist's discreet self-disclosure of affect (Maroda, 2022). For example, over those weeks of working with and through Lucinda's core wound she would sometimes enter session in a combined state of highly activated anxiety coupled with visceral freeze, the latter of which is the basis of dissociation. I often felt this as a tightness and shakiness in my own guts. When I let her know my somatic experience—that I was aware of a gripping in my gut—and that I needed us to slow down so that I could catch up with myself and be with her, she subsequently realized how she was experiencing something similar. Introducing my own somatic experience gave her more permission to be with hers. She did not ask about the personal content of my experience—I contained that—and there was no need to further self-disclose. Her tendency is to cognitively override (split off) physically felt manifestations and, thus, the feelings embedded there. My naming my experience signaled that bringing in more of her experience was possible. From there, we were able to stay directly engaged with what was immediately unfolding within, allowing us to continue the working through process.

Reflecting Again on Enactments

If one of the central tasks of the analyst is to bear, accept, and be with not knowing, then at best, for me, this will always be a practice. This book focuses on striving to conceptually understand, and at the same time show how, we might somatically apprehend the complex territory of embodied psychic life within oneself and those with whom we work. However, simultaneously cultivating a relationship with that which is subjectively unknowable gives rise to a *coniunctio*. The opposites come together and birth a sense of mystery, the mystery of the unknowable unfolding between one's self and another. For me, consciousness of the unknown serves as a guide to enter the consulting room without "memory or desire" (Bion, 1988). This state of open curiosity can give birth to everyday joys, ecstasies, and sorrows, sometimes engendering awe and sometimes moments of despair. Analytic love emerges from the challenge and surprise of navigating this territory.

This mystery is borne as I experience my bodily self in the analytic encounter. Our bodily selves are organically constructed to be semipermeable and exquisitely sensitive to the other, which I believe is a gift. The analytic encounter can be a dance—a highly complex one—but energetically a dance, nonetheless. In this dance, I am keenly vulnerable to being affected by those with whom I work, just as they are to me. There is choice as to what we do with how we are affected—be it to attune, empathize, be surely located in one's own experience distinct from the other, which allows for compassion—that is connection and separateness. In addition, there are boundaried moves toward establishing separateness, feedback, interpretation, confrontation, and, when desired or necessary, disconnection. That is the inevitability of being affected (Maroda, 2022).

At times, when experiencing psychophysical distress, awareness practices coupled with reflective inquiry enable me to turn the volume up or down on difficult feelings and sensations I am experiencing, or at least surf the waves of those experiences. In contrast, at other times, I feel I am in the midst of some alchemical reaction that is beyond my influence. Then, time reflection, meditation, movement, and consultation are factors. Sometimes, I am able to move through to deeper connection and understanding, but not in the way I might imagine. Sometimes, when I am not clear about what is happening within, what I can do is bear witness.

In personal communication, a cosmologist and dear colleague, Brian Swimme, reviewed with me what the farthest reaches of the cosmos have been telling us by the mysteries brought to us via the James Webb telescope. "In the Biblical tradition," he said, "order is imposed on chaos. But our current understanding is that chaotic violence, such as an exploding star, is *essential* for the emergence of order. A difficult truth to integrate into our lives, no doubt." The reverberations of the enactments I have described felt metaphorically like those of an exploding star, engendering a sense of shock and awe. The enactment, rather than being a disaster resulting in a misalignment for Eva and her guiding star, or for us and our work, brought a new emergent order.

Jung's words come to mind here: "For two personalities to meet is like mixing two chemical substances if there is any combination at all both are transformed" (1966/1946, para. 163).

In closing, I emphasize that this chapter is not intended to be an exhaustive accounting of the therapist's somatic experience in general, but rather to open a window onto somatically inclusive psychological thinking as to what might be experienced in the somatic dimension of the therapist's experience.

References

Ammaniti, M., & Ferrari, P. (2013). Vitality affects in Daniel Stern's thinking: A psychological and neurobiological perspective. *Infant Mental Health Journal, 34*(5), 367–375.

Bion, W. (1988). Notes on memory and desire. In E. B. Spillius (Ed.), *Melanie Klein today: Developments in theory and practice, vol. 2. Mainly practice* (pp. 17–21). London: Taylor & Frances/Routledge. First published in 1967 in *Psychoanalytic Forum, 2*, 272–273, 279–280.

Boston Change Process Study Group (BCPSG). (2013). Enactment and the emergence of new relational organization. *Journal of the American Psychoanalytic Association, 61*, 727–749.

Bromberg, P. M. (2011). *The shadow of the tsunami and the growth of the relational mind.* New York: Routledge.

Cwik, A. J. (2011). Associative dreaming: Reverie and active imagination. *Journal of Analytical Psychology, 1*, 14–36.

Eliade, M. (1964). *Shamanism: Archaic techniques of ecstasy.* W. R. Trask (Trans.). Princeton, NJ: Princeton University Press.

Fuchs, T. (2017). Intercorporeality and interaffectivity. In C. Meyer, J. Streeck, & J. S. Jordan (Eds.), *Intercorporeality: Emerging socialities in interaction, foundations of human interaction.* New York: Oxford University Press. https://doi.org/10.1093/acprof:oso/9780190210465.003.0001

Fuchs, T. & Koch, S. (2014). Embodied affectivity: On moving and being moved. *Frontiers in Psychology, 5*, 508. Pre-published online April 14, 2014. Published online June 6, 2014. https://doi.org/10.3389/fpsyg.2014.00508

Gallese, V. (2009). Mirror neurons, embodied simulation, and the neural basis of social identification. *Psychoanalytic Dialogues, 19*(5), 519–536.

———— (2012). Embodied simulation theory and intersubjectivity. Corisco Edizioni. Retrieved Dec. 27, 2023, from Corisco Edizioni.

Gallese, V., & Guerra, M. (2019). *The empathic screen: Cinema and neuroscience.* F. Anderson (Trans.). Oxford: Oxford University Press.

Halifax, J. (1990). The Shaman's initiation. *ReVision, 2*, 53–61.

Jung, C. G. (1966/1935). Principles of practical psychotherapy (1935, p. 8). In H. Read, M. Fordham, & G. Adler (Eds.). *The collected works of C. G. Jung, vol. 16: Practice of psychotherapy.* R. F. C. Hull (Trans.). Princeton, NJ: Princeton University Press.

———— (1966/1946). *The practice of psychotherapy: Essays on the psychology of the transference and other subjects.* R. F. C. Hull (Trans.). Paras 163, 358. Princeton, NJ: Princeton University Press.

Klein, M. (1952). The origins of transference. International Journal of Psychoanalysis, 33(4), 433–443.

Maroda, K. (2022). *The analyst's vulnerability.* New York, London: Routledge.

Sedgwick, D. (1994). *The wounded healer: Countertransference from a Jungian perspective.* London, New York: Routledge.

———— (2014). Jung as a pioneer of relational analysis, nwaps.org. Updated February 25, 2014, retrieved December 30, 2023.

Stern, D. N. (2018/1985). *The interpersonal world of the infant: View from psychoanalysis and developmental psychology.* New York: Basic Books.

van Löben Sels, R. (2019). *Shamanic dimensions of psychotherapy: Healing through the symbolic process.* London, New York: Routledge.

Chapter 9

The Poetics of Embodiment

In the following chapter, I will discuss how the affective life in groups is activated in an approach to Active Imagination, interchangeably known as Authentic Movement or Movement in Depth, in which the body, as experienced in stillness and movement, becomes the medium for exploration. In that practice, the containment created in oscillating phases of nonconceptual, bodily-based exploration done in silence to carefully structured periods of verbal dialogue, a highly attuned intersubjective field emerges. Within a group atmosphere such as this, participants find the emotional safety that allows for a level of emotional availability not often found in dyadic, verbal forms of therapy. As participants touch on what is most essential, new possibilities emerge, and healing unfolds.

Jung's Paradoxical Perspective on Groups in the Context of Individuation

I want first to acknowledge Jung's paradoxical perspective on groups. Jung was rather allergic to groups, and understandably so. He saw the dangers of "groupthink" play out in the horrors of the Third Reich. In addition, Jung observed that organized religion and other exclusive groups tend to degrade the spiritual, moral, and ethical attitudes of their original teachings. This led him to think that individuals, upon becoming a member of a group or sect, were less able to think or feel independently. Jung's observations caution us about the negative dynamics of groups. However, Mary Watkins (2022) pinpoints the limitations: "While understandable in the context of the rise of fascism, his distrust caused him to neglect reflection on the kinds of groups and group process that are conducive to insights rarely possible on one's own."

Jung emphasized the necessity of the individual to differentiate from the collective and group affiliation, including one's family and the social conventions of the times. Analysis, which included attending to the archetypal elements that accrue in the psyche rooted in these relationships, was the way to achieve this differentiation, and Individuation was the goal. Jungian analysis is an invitation to engage your creative unconscious. Accompanied by your analyst, you explore uncharted territory within that is rich with dreams, symbols, and archetypes unique to you. It is

DOI: 10.4324/9781003305804-10

a poetics of the psyche. Paramount to such a journey is working with wounds and obstacles of relationship, the gift of which opens you to the other and the world. Yet, Jung's concept of "Individuation" is as misunderstood as any in the Jungian lexicon. Given that it is the goal of Jungian analysis, this is problematic.

Jung attempted to correct the misunderstandings of the concept of Individuation as an individual's inner work done in isolation solely for the sake of themselves (Watkins, 2022). Jung wrote:

> Individuation is only possible with people and through people. You must realize that you are a link in a chain. You are not an electron suspended somewhere in space or aimlessly drifting through the cosmos. You are part of an atomic structure, and that atomic structure is part of a molecule which, with others, builds up a body.
> … Individuation does not shut one out from the world but gathers the world to oneself.
>
> Jung (1972/1954, para. 432)

Interdependence, Interaffectivity, and the Web of Life

Now, more than ever, clarification of the concept of Individuation is crucial because nothing is more essential for our survival than the recognition of ourselves as part of the chain of life. It is paramount to develop the capacity to negotiate our interdependence—with each other and the more-than-human-others with whom we are utterly interdependent.

While Jung's intuition, brilliance, and prescience were remarkable, some Jungian analysts and thinkers struggle with the contradictions, at times regressive and offensive, on one side of Jung's often paradoxical viewpoints toward issues such as groups, Individuation, gender, race, and ethnicity.

Many work to confront and update these issues. Mary Watkins (2022) does so when she invites us to see through the normalization of oppressive structures and relationships, partly through the recovery of historical memory. In the Active Imagination practice of Movement in Depth, the body serves as the portal of access to engage the implicit layers of these historical memories.

The oppression Watkins refers to, once internalized, is often directed toward one's body. This may manifest in an attempt to dominate the body—how it looks, what it can and cannot do—and by eradicating the emotional pain the body bears. When we are blind to these inner dynamics, the unprocessed affect leaks into the collective and, at times, is actively projected onto others. Forging a bond with our bodily experience is fundamental to relating to the multiplicity of selves within each of us to gain greater awareness of implicit patterns in our relationships with others. It is the act of making conscious the somatic unconscious. Turning toward and holding the opposites within ourselves is the basis of the inner and outer democracy Don Kalsched (2023) so eloquently orients us toward in our work as depth psychotherapists.

In this time, with the existential threat of climate catastrophe, many desperately want to cultivate a sustainable world and are hungry for collaborative interdependence. The practice of being together in a bodily-based, psychologically savvy, and non-conceptually saturated unfolding experience, I believe, offers a small but important contribution toward the potential inherent in the life of a conscious collective.

This contribution is based on the profundity of interaffectivity (Fuchs, 2017)—particularly its positive pole. In addition to Jung, many others have written about the negative pole using terms like emotional contagion, infection, and absenting. Understanding the neurological basis of interaffectivity might help navigate the complexities of group life. Mirror neurons, adaptive isolators, and the capacity for mimicking are part of our neurological makeup and inform us about what is occurring in another. In review, mirror neurons are activated when we see another move with intent. Adaptive isolators are those neurological mechanisms that allow us to move in sync with one another without the rational effort that would require working out each distinct movement and the vitality and rhythm intrinsic to that movement. We can readily bring this to mind via experiences of dancing or learning a new sport. Interaffectivity emerges as these basic biological structures couple with embodied affectivity—we are moved by and move with others (BCPSG, 2018).

Because it is a biological given, there is value in consciously mitigating the hurtful and destructive aspects of the negative pole of interaffectivity while cultivating the positive pole.

Foundational to addressing the negative pole is recognizing and working with projection to reintegrate shadow material. This is fundamental in the practice of Movement in Depth. In what follows, I will describe one approach to bringing conscious attention to how an affective, resonant, and responsive field is constellated through the practice of Movement in Depth. There is no other situation in which I have come to so directly experience the African concept of *Ubuntu* (*I am because you are*) than in this practice. It has helped me to recognize this truth in those relationships I find the most challenging, as well as those that are the most intimate.

A Brief History of Authentic Movement/ Movement in Depth

Focusing on Interaffectivity in This Form of Group Work

First, I will give a brief account of the history of Authentic Movement and describe the practice. Then, I will weave immediate first-person accounts of individual and interactive experiences alongside theoretical narratives to portray the nonverbal unfolding of body-based experience. As verbal expression does emerge in this practice, you will see that it does so in language much more akin to poetry than linear prose.

While there is literature on the dyadic practice of Authentic Movement (Adler 1999/1972; Adler 1999/1976; Adler 2002; Chodorow, 1999/1977; Chodorow,

1999/1984; Chodorow, 1991; Fleischer, 2023; Holifield, 2007; Musicant, 2007; Pallaro, 1999, 2007; Stromsted, 2007; Wasson, 2007; Wyman-McGinty, 2007), and its profound contribution to facilitating and understanding the psychological nuances of embodiment, less has been written regarding group work (Adler, 2002; Adler, Morrissey & Sager, 2022). In this chapter, I will focus on interaffectivity in this form of group work because I believe it offers an important perspective on groups with applicable value in our current times.

A large international community now engages in this practice rooted in Mary Whitehouse's courageous and determined intent to express what she knew from her experience about psyche's bodily basis. In addition to working with Charlotte Selver, Whitehouse studied with Mary Wigman and Martha Graham. She went on to teach at UCLA, the Jung Institute of Los Angeles, and privately. Her first paper, "Creative Expression in Physical Movement is Language without Words," in which she discussed her approach, was written c.1956.[1] Beginning in the late 1970s, I immersed myself in the practice over a five-year period while apprenticing with a psychologist, Edward Maupin, whose work focused on embodiment. Maupin had studied with Mary Whitehouse at UCLA. Following this, I spent another decade in New York City studying and teaching with Alton Wasson. This contributed to an ever-deepening appreciation for the elegance of this noninterpretive, self-directed, yet fully relational approach to understanding embodiment. Authentic Movement/Movement in Depth offered an immediacy to embodied self-knowledge and continually opened me to new possibilities. I found that to engage in the practice was to step into an alternative state of consciousness, a different quality of time, one more akin to Kairos than Chronos. There is something of an ego death in crossing the threshold and surrendering to what is unknown, a fundamental aspect of this practice. Everything that occurred was always a surprise, which was partly why this was so intriguing.[2] And these surprises changed me for the better. This was true whether I entered intending to work with muddled psychophysical pain rooted in personal history, or open to exploring the unfolding moment. I knew then that this would remain an ongoing current in my personal and professional practice, and I wanted to learn all I could. Intent on pursuing Jungian Analytic training, I moved from New York City to San Francisco, where I knew I could incorporate study with Janet Adler and Joan Chodorow, two of Mary Whitehouse's primary students, with my analytic training. These women further developed the practice, becoming the cornerstones of a far-reaching community of practitioners.

It was in the mid-1960s when Mary Whitehouse boldly transformed her dance studio into a space for something other than dance to occur (Adler et al., 2022, p. 2). Having embarked on the inward journey of psyche through a Jungian Analysis, she was compelled to explore how the psyche unfolded in the body. In her movement studio, she sat to the side of the space, sometimes in silence and sometimes using prompts, to guide students in discovering a way to be in their bodies from a more inwardly sourced place. Focusing on process rather than outer form, she sought to elicit that something that occurred when dance truly came alive and when aliveness, in all its up-and-down variations, can be felt to emanate from within (Whitehouse, 1999/1956).

Engaging the Implicit Realm in Psychotherapy Leads to Deep Change

This something other-than-dance parallels the something other-than-interpretation in psychoanalysis that the BCSPG honed in on—the largely bodily-based realm of relational experiencing in which change in psychotherapy occurs (detailed in Chapter 5).[3] Similarly, those in the Zen community understood that Charlotte Selver's work with Sensory Awareness elicited that something other than the experience of formal meditation practice, a something that had similarities with meditation but could occur in formal meditation as well as in activities of everyday life. The realm of overlap in these approaches is the immediacy of knowing that arises when awareness is brought to unfolding bodily-based, nonconceptual experience.

Eugene Gendlin's research (1962, 1995, 1997, 2017) also revealed how contacting this implicit realm in psychotherapy leads to more profound therapeutic change. He extended this study to include the significance of implicit experience in creative thinking. He sometimes used the terms "dipping" and "crossing." "Dipping" describes purposefully attending to the private bodily-based, subjective space as a source of knowing and creativity, and "crossing" to the verbal explication. He understood that explication changes or furthers what is found in the implicit realm, leading to renewed dipping, another change step, and more new experiences (Gendlin,1995). He illuminated how words *further* one's direct subjective experience rather than the idea that words should precisely *describe* one's direct experience. Gendlin's dipping and crossing aptly describes the cyclical process of moving followed by dialogue in Movement in Depth. It is also descriptive of the dialogue that unfolds between the mover and the witness(es). The carefully languaged dialogue allows what has happened in the movement sessions and what unfolds in the telling to come further into conscious awareness. It is a way of bringing the body, the nonconceptual world, into language. The dialogue stays tethered to the inquiry of how we make sense of the treasure of nonconceptual experience without foreclosing on it with words. The emphasis in the dialogue practice is to linger with what the body knows, and what more it comes to know, through attentive listening and reflection. When spoken within the crafted practice, the words attempt to express what is, along with what just occurred—dipping and crossing between the somatically informed, nonconceptual, and verbal worlds.

Mary Whitehouse's early explorations, teachings, presentations, and writings (in Pallaro, 1999) seeped up like the headwaters of a river—waters that upswell at the spring, slowly forming a stream that gains momentum as it is fed by other seeps and sources, in time becoming a coursing river. This current flowed into the mainstream of Jungian Analysis, shifting perspectives. The significance of the body, highlighted by contemporary trauma studies, infant research, the BCSPG, and neuroscience, has added force to the current. Whitehouse's contributions mark the early shifts of perspective in the Jungian world, from a predominantly conceptual and image-based orientation to an embodied, affect-oriented approach to the clinical and archetypal realm. Jung perceived the entwining of body and psyche, and regarded emotion as the primary motivating factor of the psyche—including archetype as affect and image—yet this has not always been operationally apparent in the literature, training, or practice of a Jungian approach.

The Practice of Authentic Movement

Authentic Movement (Pallaro, 1999) is a profoundly simple process in which one or more active participants, in the presence of one or more witnesses, turn their attention inward and attend to unfolding sensations and impulses toward movement or stillness and, if present, arising of affects. In responding to these inner promptings, other ongoing inner stirrings of psyche arise, such as memories, images, dreams, and intermittent narratives, which continually influence the subjective experience of what unfolds. The emphasis is on attending to the felt sense in the body and leaning into nonconceptual experience as a guide. As we soften reliance on conceptual understanding and instead focus awareness on the inwardly experienced body, less familiar ways of perceiving are set in motion. As impulses to move or be in stillness emerge, one can choose to follow one of these, or none. Either way, recognizing one's choice and carefully tracking what unfolds is paramount. As elements of psychological content arise, close tracking of bodily-based experience relinks these to their implicit roots. This fosters a felt sense of embodiment.

Settling into this inward realm is often felt as coming home, a claiming and embodying of an awareness of self. Awareness of self expands when cultivating the felt sense of the internal space of the body. Openly inquiring in this way tends to loosen and soften the tensional field of the body, and awareness of associated feeling states comes into focus (Fuchs 2020). In the practice, this unfolds in a relational context. Being seen by an attentive other helps us see ourselves more clearly. This further contributes to loosening the binds of singular identification (merger) with any one part of the self. This is an intriguing phenomenon—the simple act of purposeful attention to sense, and to feel one's body with an attitude of open curiosity in the presence of an attentive witness can facilitate disidentification with singular self-states. Such an inquiry might simply explore "who am I here?" Tracking one's bodily-felt sensations, emotions, and imagination, in turn, activates an inner witness. The inner witness then learns to track further the multiplicity of self-experiences, which paves the way for developing an awareness of the one within who is aware.

Authentic Movement becomes a laboratory to study and experience how this happens not just in one individual, but in other group members at the same time. Witnesses purposefully attune to those who are movers. Movers become moving witnesses; that is, movers, if desired, purposefully attune to others moving in the circle. With this, the interaffective field—the awareness of embodied affective resonance and discordance—becomes highly sensitized.

Movement periods ranging from five to 45 minutes are followed by periods of silence during which one can choose to silently reflect, write, or draw to map and further know their profoundly intimate, subjective experience. As I mentioned, careful dialogue between the mover(s) and witness(es) follows. The emphasis is on allowing meaning to emerge from direct experience. This may incorporate the direct experience of the immediacy of relationship with the witness(es), the specific unfolding felt experiences in the body, including the actual movements, or the felt urge or pattern of movement, including those that are so subtle or inward that they are imperceptible to the witness. Accompanying affects, images, and memories can be spoken if one chooses to do so as they emerge into awareness. Some have likened the individual work to Freudian-based free association—yet here, the whole person includes the personal and collective unconscious as well as the body, sensing, feeling, and imagining—and the floor is the couch (Castle, 2001).

As a mover works, the witness sits to the side and carefully tracks what she sees—the active mover's specific movements, including the outwardly expressive as well as subtle affective expressions, such as those made visible by facial expression, breath, sighs, sounds, and other muscular actions and patterns. The inner attention of the witness is similar to the mover's—attending carefully to what unfolds within, staying closely tethered to somatic experience. A guiding principle for both mover and witness is cultivating a non-interpretive, nonjudgmental attitude. The foundation of the witness practice is to notice what you "see" (a special kind of soft, focused attention of seeing *and* sensing), and how you are affected. Through disciplined practice, witnesses foster reflective awareness of personal projection and the ability to contain these and work with their psychological material as it arises in order to be present in themselves and for the mover. Once in dialogue with the mover, the witness's response will be offered without interpretation, judgment, or criticism. When words are spoken, the witness also speaks in the first-person present tense.

Usually, the mover speaks first, though this may change in group work as trust is established. A great deal of attention is paid to bringing the experience of the body to language. Speaking in the first-person present tense, whether talking about the experience of having moved or what is unfolding in the moment of speaking, brings forward the psychic reality of that experience. Not unlike a dream, it is considered as a living psychic reality rather than an event gone by.

Authentic or Inauthentic, Movement or Stillness?

Mary Whitehouse referred to the practice with various terms, including Authentic Movement, Movement in Depth, and The Moving Imagination. While the international community has adopted the name "Authentic Movement," I have found this gives rise to an intellectual quandary of what constitutes authentic versus inauthentic movement, causing confusion about the right or wrong way to practice. I prefer "Movement in Depth," as Mary Whitehouse sometimes used, or my long-hand version, "Being with the Body as Experienced in Movement and Still-ness." Though a mouthful, the latter softens yet another polarization that some-times arises between movement and stillness. I will use the names interchangeably.

The international community also refers to the one who is not the formal "wit-ness" as the "mover." I find this a source of confusion for those unfamiliar with the practice. In actual practice, the active participant who is not the "witness" might not "move" but rather enter deep states of stillness. When stillness is explored with awareness, there is inevitably movement, such as breathing and heartbeat. Those unfamiliar with the practice who hear the term "mover" imagine that one has to *move*, and, moreover, move creatively! Again, a polarity is constellated be-tween moving and stillness, and between creative and ordinary expression. Some of my most extraordinary experiences in practicing have come from entering deep stillness.

"Active participant" is also a misleading term for the "mover" because the wit-ness does not outwardly move, yet is intently active—tracking the others' move-ment and their own interoceptive and affective experience (Adler, 1999/1987; Chodorow, 1999/1986). For now, I will continue to use the familiar terms with the hope that this explanation clarifies for those unfamiliar with the work.

The Body as the Medium of Experience in Active Imagination: Authentic Movement

A Focus on Interaffectivity

Twelve seasoned psychotherapists with experience with Authentic Movement,[4] have gathered at Green Gulch Zen Center, just north of San Francisco.[5] We will be here for a three-day Authentic Movement Retreat. It is early morning as we enter the circular space of the Yurt to practice. Nestled amongst towering euca-lyptus and redwoods, the yurt sits just yards away from the creek that carves its way down the headlands and through Green Gulch. When first erected, the yurt provided Charlotte Selver a place to teach Sensory Awareness. One of the pioneers in the Somatics field, she brought her simple yet profound practice to the Zen Buddhist community here more than 60 years ago. Her teachings emphasized the body sensed and experienced rather than the body that is conceived and performed. She taught until she was 102 and died at her home just down the gulch from here. Her work influenced a great many in the field of psychology during that remark-able period. I feel a sense of honor and belonging, knowing she taught here. Mary Whitehouse, who pioneered the practice of Authentic Movement, was strongly in-fluenced by Charlotte Selver. I studied here in the yurt with Janet Adler, one of Mary's primary students, for nearly a decade. A peer group, of which I am a mem-ber, was formed when Janet stepped down from teaching us. We have continued to meet here in the yurt for Authentic Movement Retreats for over 20 years. Today,

I will be facilitating a newly constellated group. We will continue focusing on being with the body as experienced, now within the context of depth psychotherapy.

As the wind rises and falls, the yurt responds. The semi-permeable boundary of the skin of the yurt, of our own skin—between inside and out—is palpable. It is early spring. Songbirds fill the Gulch with their music. It is easy to distinguish the song of the newborn from the adult. The unbridled joy of the fledgling's song proclaims life renewed. The adults create a sublime harmony as the beauty of the melancholic, flute-like call and response of the hermit thrush mixes with tanagers, warblers, ravens, and red tails. Occasionally, a eucalyptus pod drops onto the top of the yurt with a loud crack. At that moment, its sharp fragrance enters the open windows. Now and then, the wind sweeps up-canyon, carrying the sound of ocean waves rolling in at Muir Beach. These other-than-human beings are essential participants and are every bit as important as the women in the circle.

As the facilitator, I tap the large ancient Tibetan Bowl with a wooden mallet. Its sound announces the beginning of the first round of a 30-minute movement session on our third and final day of retreat.

The Green Gulch Retreat

Third Morning

After two days of sorting and moving into and through present psychophysical entanglements, inquiries, and wanderings, a sense of arriving at an edge is present this morning. What will unfold on this final day of the retreat? Much has been stirred. How will our embodied psyches respond? Will there be a reconciliation within each individual of the pain and tension of unresolved inquiries and opened wounds? As we begin, I speak to the group about the Japanese practice of *Kintsugi*—honoring, rather than hiding, the cracks and breakage of a ceramic vessel by repairing it with gold. In this process, the vessel becomes even more valuable and beautiful. In analogy, our life is a Golden Path of Rejoining—our consciousness is the gold that fills the breakage and gaps generated by life's challenges, and reconnects us with ourselves, each other, and the more-than-human others.

In our first practice of this morning we begin outside, spread along the creek and surrounding meadow. I ring the bell. Each woman first witnesses, in silence, an element of the natural world. Following this, each woman allows themself to be witnessed by that elemental force for a few more minutes.[6]

When we re-enter the yurt, participants bring how they have been affected by the more-than-human others, part of our greater conscious collective, in their practice as they move and witness. After a round of moving inside the yurt, we gather to share the words emerging from the morning's practice. These verbal offerings arise from the direct experience of witnessing and moving outside, as well as of witnessing and moving inside the yurt while further incorporating the time outside.

Participants' First-person Narratives

A Witness Outside
> *I see you standing so tall I cannot see the end of your long limbs*
> *gently swinging in a breeze, reaching toward the sky.*
> *I see you in a group of relatives, but you are not originally from here.*
> *I see you right on the edge—the ground drops in front of you.*
> *I notice right at the base of your lean, vibrant body a small stump,*
> *attached to you,*
> *lifeless.*
> *As I see your lifelessness, I remember the pull to collapse yesterday when,*
> *as I moved, I felt the weight of a dead child in my arms, not mine but ours—*
> *the one killed by the police, the one who fell to his accidental death too young,*
> *the one waiting too long in her crib for a mother who doesn't come.*

Now Moving
> *I remember the invitation in our practice today is to notice the familiar impulse, inhibit the familiar response, and track what happens inside. The impulse is so strong to drop to the ground, but I stand rather than act on the impulse. I hold the heaviness of the lifeless child. A tear forms on my cheek, then another. I am moved, moved to bring the child into my womb.*

Witnessing Again
> *Now, I look more carefully at the dead part of you and see,*
> *a splash of green fanning out from a ridged sheath, a delicate bright green stem, with open leafy arms topped by a cluster of red dots, gray ripples growing through the cracks of the dead surface—each thriving—*
> *the deadness now hosting your own unique aliveness.*

My Witnessing Inside
> *In the beginning, five movers, with their eyes closed, move from the circle's periphery*
> *toward the center of the yurt. Above is a circular skylight.*
> *The soft morning light filters in. The movers now trace its circumference,*
> *situating themselves in a quadrant within this center of soft light facing toward one another:*
> *One mover stands with hands behind her back.*
> *The one across from her stands also with her hands behind her back.*

One mover sits, her left arm extended, and her palm open.
The one near her lies with her left arm extending above her head.
One mover stands with both hands, palms open and out, as does another
who is quite near.
As their witness, I see hands move in synchrony, sensing and being sensed
by that which is invisible.
I feel I am in the presence of an unfolding ritual.

At times like this, the choreography that unfolds and is seen by witnesses, though completely unseen and unplanned by the movers, is often stunningly beautiful in its symmetry, counterpoints of disjunction, timing, return to symmetry, and closure.

A Mover
Lying on my right side, I imagine myself in Germany, where my mother was
raised. I think of my family still there. I imagine I am at my aunt's house, in
the forest. I remember the special connection I feel to the land there. A long-
ing stirs in me even though, when there, I feel the tension of their judgment.
I recall the way they walk in the land as if they belong in it.
I, as her Witness, ask,
What happens in your body that lets you know this?

The Mover Responds
I see my mother and feel a tingling presence in the center of my chest.
There is warmth in my hips and thighs as I remember how she picks plums
and casually eats them as she walks, leaving no flesh on the pit. I salivate;
my throat is expectant, hungry. I feel blessed—in this place, the fruit belongs
to anyone who walks this path. Again, I feel longing and solitude, wavering
between all these.
The heel of my foot lands in another mover's hand. I sense this as support
that needs nothing from me . . . Now, the other's fingers lightly tap my foot.
I understand that her fingers are saying goodbye and that it is okay.
I don't know how I know this, this sense that the other mover is saying
more than goodbye. Her fingers brush and gently tap, tap, tap my foot like
raindrops; she gives it time and stays with that motion. I'm reminded of being
a mother, preparing my baby for some transition by letting him know what's
coming next. She's tapping my foot with her fingers, and I know this means,
"I am leaving soon." I marvel that fingers alone could communicate this. She

is not rushed. She is not staying just to avoid disappointing me. She cares about what I am feeling. I wonder how I know. I relish this; it's new.[7] *I don't feel ashamed or confused about making someone stay. It is time for her to go, and she is staying with the going, so that I can get used to it. When she does leave, I feel prepared, and I know her leaving is not because of something I have done.*

I like that way of moving away—barely perceptible yet still moving.

Another Witness Speaks to the Mover whose Hand Caught the Heel

I see you, your hand cradling another's foot. I hear you speak of sending a message through touch that communicates that you will be taking your leave soon. I am touched by the love and care in this gesture. I remember my grandmother, who passed away just a couple of months ago, and how, in the last few years of her life, all of her actions said, "I love you, I will be saying goodbye soon." I feel the love in your gesture, the gift of my grandmother's tending, and am deeply touched and grateful.

Two of the previous entries express the experience of being in a land that is not the one where they or their ancestors were raised, and the sometimes fatal pain of being othered. The reverberations of a change in one's outer lived place live in the inner place of the body. One participant speaks of the effect of displacement of another species. This will be echoed later, at the end of this morning's session, by yet another mover as she finds her body echoing what she sees in another species that has been displaced to this land.

A Mover's Poem Arising from Bringing Her Witnessing Outside into Movement Inside

Be Like a Plum Tree
Be like a plum tree
Impossibly beautiful
Perfect little green leave
Innumerable
Shimmering
Dancing
In sunlight and shadow
Like a thousand tiny tickling fingers
Be like a plum tree
When the mind calls you to other things

Be like a plum tree
Be gentle
Be strong
Be rooted
Be wild
Be like a plum tree
On the edge of a marsh
Cattails and horsetails
Swaying in light
Be like a plum tree
Moss, lichen, scars, roots.
Be like a plum tree
Be shelter
Be safety
Be food
Be home
Be like a plum tree
Be slow
Be quiet
Be still
Be like a plum tree
Stand rooted
Reach up for sun
Be like a plum tree

I Witness

You stand in your full length. I see your face—the muscles there are soft and open. Your arms extend down, palms open and out. You sway ever so slightly as a flower does to receive the sun—your body turns, your hands turn, your fingers quietly and delicately flicker. I imagine you are taking in the nourishment that is touching you, entering you. You do this for a long time. Now another mover leans into your leg. Her head near your thigh. You stroke her hair intimately. I imagine her as your daughter, now I imagine you as a daughter, and now I imagine you as a daughter to yourself. I feel a gentle tingling in my chest and an opening that spreads and deepens.

A Nearby Mover Speaks of Becoming the Leaning Tree

I am a mover who remembers the eucalyptus tree I just witnessed outside the yurt. I stretch and explore the movements of my shoulders and back and imagine the meeting point of limbs and trunk.

I remember an oak tree outside my home. The one that we call "the leaning oak." I lie on my side and shape my body to mimic the shape of our leaning oak friend. I stretch and explore the space with one arm branch while being supported by my other arm branch.

I play with the possibilities of leaning.

I remember all the beings protected, nourished, and housed by our leaning oak friend. My leaning hip and head find yet another body to my right. I feel their hand gently touch my head. I play with leaning away and towards this other, which I imagine as another tree.

As my branches explore this space, I think about the diversity within this group, the idea of strength, how my neurodivergence is intertwined with my divergent and varying physical needs—the various ways that my body–mind diverges. My body knows there isn't just one way to be strong. I feel appreciation for the diversity within our oak forest of movers.

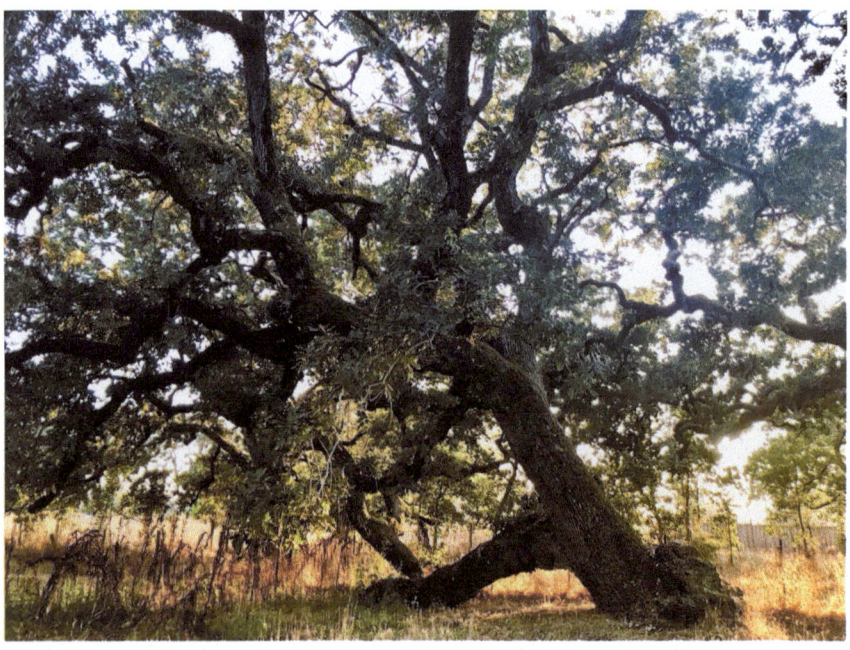

Figure 9.1 The Leaning Tree (Photograph by Mover who Becomes the Leaning Tree, with permission)

I Witness the Mover Who Speaks of Becoming the Leaning Tree
   I hear you speak of sensing, through the palms of your hands, the outer ecosystem, and then as you place your hand on your own chest, your inner ecosystem. You speak of how, because of your neurodivergence, this is essential to how you come to know the world.
   As you describe the nuance of your sensual perception of that which is housed in the tree you describe and imagine yourself to be, an unexpected sense of surprise comes over me. As if I have traveled to a foreign land and am awakened to something I had not known before. Later, I see you lean into another mover's leg. She gently touches your hair.

Neurodiversity

This mover finds that the practice of Movement in Depth allows her the freedom to be herself. To lean into her unique gifts, strengths, and resources. These include her keen sensitivity to the environment, liberty to adjust closeness and distance with others, and the ability to develop and be with distinct realms of sensory perception.

Participants' First-person Narratives (continued)

I Witness the Mover Who Discovers She, Too, Is a Perfectly Imperfect Offering
   I hear you speak of the beauty of the eucalyptus tree you witnessed outside, alongside struggling with the tension of your judgment of it.[8] *You move into the circle and are contacted by one mover and then another. I hear you describe how, as you receive this touch, you are filled—infused with acceptance—the ecstatic liberation of self-acceptance of your perfectly imperfect offering. The words of this morning's invocation echo within you now: "there is a crack in everything. My whole body is pulsing with the light coming in."*

Interaffectivity

As the group drops ever more deeply into this realm of purposeful silence and into the feeling body, the conceptual world of words loosens its distinct edges. Aspects of the nonverbal world, often hidden, begin to emerge. In this process, both mover and witness cultivate a highly attuned self-reflective practice of embodied response to their inner world. A powerful and heightened interaffective field emerges between individual movers moving together, between movers and witnesses, and between individual witnesses. The practice is a relational meditation. The work is carefully crafted to create felt psychological and physical safety, allowing the freedom to explore the vast spectrum of unfolding inner and outer territory. Once verbal dialogue begins, it can feel uncanny how one individual mover's work echoes or furthers another's, sometimes through affect and sometimes content.

Third Afternoon

A Witness Beholds the Inside Space of the Yurt

The initiation bell ricochets into an intricate web, creating overlapping layers of sound inside the yurt.

I honor my reluctance to move and, instead, compose my witness self. I gather my fractured attention from distant places by tuning into my senses one by one to decrease my mind's spikey fray. I oscillate between my own external and internal sensing and attune to deeper layers of presence with the movers.

As I witness the movers open to the unfolding emergent presence within and around them, I observe the shielded sheath surrounding my own vulnerability soften and dissipate.

A Mover Speaks

Deep fatigue invites me to surrender even more.

I enter standing, knowing I am part of this collective body.

I hear the sound of footfalls on the floor. My left hand calls in response, becoming a steady beating heart, opening and closing.

I sink into my right hip, hinging this joint with deep care and appreciation, inviting strength into the soft tissues. I stand invoking the dancing Shiva. I am still but so alive. I feel Shiva's strength and sensuous grace. I am grateful for his presence as I descend, slowly, to the earth. And now, again, fatigue invites me to surrender further.

I hear other movers near me, aware that I have yet to make physical contact with another. Curiosity and longing arise simultaneously. Will I find someone? Will someone find me? I lay in rest, and a forearm arrives in my right hand. Such soft skin, it almost feels translucent, this flesh, this forearm flesh draped gently over bone. Another hand finds my left toes, then sole of foot. This touch linking us three feels so nourishing. I am grounded and connected now. I feel at home in myself, in this circle, in this community, in this collective body.

A Standing Mover Speaks

I.

I am the one who walks.

I find my way to the center of the room, guided by the way the light feels on my face. This light has been with me all day, leading the way, outside, inward, inside outward.

I allow myself to be touched by the light. I invite in the light.

Standing upright, still, legs softly straight, I am solid on the ground.

I stretch up and up, arch back, towards the light.

I feel my opening; I feel my edge.

I return.

Standing upright, still, legs softly straight, I am more solid on the ground.

I find a rhythm of swell and return.

I swell and return.

Each cycle, I become more rooted, more solid on the ground.

II.

I am the one who is still.

Another mover bumps my leg, abrupt, sudden, and the reverberations move through me, shock waves of sensation and vibration. With each wave, I become aware of how deeply connected and solid I am.

III.

I am the one at the center.

I grow and tend and feel the reverberations, finding new rhythm, one that shakes and starts.

I am moving the earth.

I am the one who moves the earth.

I am at the center.

I am solid.

I feel enormous.

I am full of sensation.

The ground is no ground I know. I am forming it from my feet; it becomes the ground as I move.

The stillness I feel is golden.

A Witness Calls Back to Standing Woman
I am the one who sees you standing still, tall, and erect
at the very center,
feet strongly rooted,

body upright,
   undeniably here.
   These words wash over me—
   The center CAN hold!

Standing Woman Responds
   "The center can hold." These words reverberate through me in a new way. I feel this truth held in the empty space of the circle, faces of each mover and witness lit by the light. I swell and return, swell and return, swell and return.

I Witness Standing Woman
   I see you standing. It seems an invisible force lifts you upward, and another grounds you and links you to earth. As I see you, you dwell in the in-between—in your body—with a quality of certainty.
   Your torso, chest, and heart lift slightly, tilting upward. Something like light enters you. I see you absorb this light and let it pass through. I recall the feminine forms depicted in Cycladic sculpture, positioned as I see you—with sublime ease—as if communicating with that which emanates from below to above.

The Non-verbal Dimension of the Numinous

In this practice, the intent is to stay close to the bone—that is, to the immediacy of the nonconceptual experience of embodiment. Sometimes, in stillness and sometimes while moving, numinous states emerge, such as that occurring with this mover. The practice guidelines are to be with the direct experience of the nonverbal dimension of numinous energies as they arise. We lean into this direct experience and linger with what the body knows—the bodily-felt experience—rather than conceptually naming or narrative associations to the archetype. As it unfolds, the direct experience "reverberates and works its effect" on the individuals and the group as a whole.

In these movement sessions, the archetypal energies of death and rebirth that emanate throughout the natural world, especially that of the Tree of Life, Death, and Rebirth, rippled through individuals and the collective body. In the morning session, the child motif—representing potential, experienced as the loss of potential (life) is followed by its unexpected re-emergence. In the afternoon session, the "Maker of the World" embodied as Shiva emerged, followed by collapse and then surrender, leading to re-emergence through connections that gave birth to belonging. The Maker of the World emerges again, in female form embodied by another mover, Standing Woman, from whose feet the ground forms, emanated a palpable numinosity within the shared space of the yurt. These energies are at work in the group as it holds and navigates the dynamic bodily-felt affects of destruction and grief, the arising of divergent forms of strength, and, all the while, the feminine principle, is deep at work, connecting and supporting in entirely unexpected ways.

A Woman Witnessing

I see the movers, one standing tall across from me, several stretched on the floor, and several crouching at different heights in different stances. There is a harmony in this human landscape, in the geometry of this circle in this yurt tucked in the trees on the mountain slope near the ocean. Witnessing, I feel a tender sense of "being with," a sacredness, deep grounding in my base, my bones.

The space calls to me, and my body hears. My mind hesitates. What is my purpose in entering the circle? I am listening to my body.

Now She Becomes a Mover and a Moving Witness

I am gleefully rolling through what was an empty space. Now it feels like I am here in service; maybe I can contribute, maybe I am needed in some way. I stop in the center with the carpet seam just to my left; I can feel it with my hands.

I am lying face down. I sense a tallness nearby. My outstretched right-hand brushes what feels like the fingertips of a mover's hand. I feel suddenly part of a three-dimensional geometric puzzle, and I have a place in it. I smile at this. With my arm outstretched, the mover's fingers are very soft and move gently with mine. I feel gentleness in me as we lightly make contact. I now notice the feeling in my stomach as I ask myself if I am moved to match the mover or find my own rhythm. And will I stay or go?

My left hand sweeps to the side and discovers another mover who makes a sound that to me sounds like welcome and relief. I am touched and interested as I touch this mover with my left hand. Our hands grasp each other. My right hand is still gently meeting the touch of gentle fingertips. The left-hand mover is touching me firmly, and I am firm there too. Stretched between, my body is in balance with these different ways of being. When it is time to say goodbye to the gentle hand mover, I leave with care. I tap a farewell with a tiny touch of my fingertips.

Leaving, I swim into myself at the edge of this circle. When I hear the bell, I feel well-used and content. I am grateful.

I Witness Gentle Hand Mover

I am the one who sees you arriving in the center, you bump into Standing mover's legs—she is so firmly standing that the force of your bumping does not disturb her. Now you lay down. I see your hands begin to tap your fore-head energetically. The tapping seems to grow in force. I am uncertain but begin to imagine that this tapping is an intervention, opening the energetic flow through your whole body.

Like a great redwood tree, another mover rolls through the field to the center. I sense she exudes generosity, and this fills my being with awe. She stops near you. She seems to sense your presence. Her two fingers find your two fingers. When the two of you make contact, it is as if I can see a current flow through your body, bringing coherence to the energetic flow within you—I see this in the quickening of your skin's texture, the awakening of a flow in your movement that now subtly but surely courses through your whole body, where before was a stillness in some of your segments and joints.

Now, you and the other mover who was touching your hand part. She stays in the connection with the mover who is on her other side. You are on your fore-legs, torso upright. You hinge deep in your hip joints, your torso comes forward to the floor, your arms extended and sweep the floor as you straighten your torso, bringing your arms up high. This gesture repeats. To me, your movement appears to be the ancient movement of prostration. Later, as your witness, I say to you, I imagine you move in a way that you know and which is very old.

When the time comes to speak, words are not present for you; your face and eyes express this through soft, open contact when you complete your movement. Perhaps words are even more distant, given that English is not your mother tongue. You echo the word "old." There is a quiet that seems to fill the space amongst us all. I sense it as reverence.

The Gentle Hand Mover Finds Words

I close my eyes. I hear the space calling me. My ears don't listen, but my body does. I am crawling. The floor drags my arms and legs deep into the land. I am crawling toward the sea of movers. I meet a mover's hard body and my body stops. I'm lying on the well where two doctors cut my genitals. The nucleus has a long tail like a lizard and is plucked out of my womb. It exits very naturally, as if it were taking a key out of a doorway. Am I taken away or open? I can feel my uterus breathing the earth.

My hands tap my head. My hands inform me that I am alive, and re-peated actions connect my body with my land, and a deep well whose end is unknown. Many babies holding their new-born bloody umbilical cord smell bloody. Are these all my babies? Where am I now, and what do I experience? My hands start tapping the floor. As tapping continues, the feeling of tapping penetrates my whole body. My body, as Bodhisattva,[9] is full of mercy and pain at the same time. Tapping indicates that these two are in my body at the same time. They experience bloody red and purple wailing together in a heart where pain is swirling. I repeat over and over that my body is shattered and then brought back together. It is the movement of my body as a child, not the current body. I was a person out of the world and a person who didn't belong and shouldn't belong. Borderlands.

My eyes are closed, but my body feels the approach of another's body. My two fingers look for the other mover's finger like an antenna. I find the movement of those two fingers that connect my world to the rest of the world and move together. The other mover's fingers take me to the deep blood and milk in me. I feel electricity flowing throughout my body. I am me and a Bodhisattva at the same time, and a person who embodies compassion until the end. I go back a long time. Back when I was something before me. My hips and limbs move repeatedly, connecting with the earth and hearing the sound of the sky. My womb opens the door and transforms all of this. My womb sings. My womb is stained with blood and makes milk. The movement of other Moving Witnesses becomes calm, and I am reborn in the circle. This circle is the mover's womb that conceived me. I am newly born in the womb, inside and outside of the circle.

Interaffectivity and Ceremony

When the kind of deep intimacy that can be known through dyadic analytic work expands into a disciplined group process in which the foundation of the exploration is nonverbal experience, something akin to ceremony or ritual unfolds. We enter an intimacy with life's unfolding. Being with the felt interior of our own body fosters intimacy with self and, when with others similarly attuned, intimacy with others.

A mover's response to the unseen gestures of other movers reverberates between them. This can be visually apparent or illuminated later in the verbal sharing. Often, the gesture of one mover, whether there is contact or not, is reciprocated by another mover or movers—a reciprocity that gives rise to the next emergent thing between the two. The healing unfolding in these unplanned and unexpected interactions can seem uncanny. As movers interact with eyes closed, contact is sometimes part of that unfolding (if this occurs, it is within the safe guidelines of the practice and always with choice). That contact may be as simple as bumping into another. It might be a hand that extends purposefully (with eyes closed) toward a mover whose tears or distress are audible.

> The communication or comprehension of gestures comes about through the reciprocity of my intentions and the gestures of others, of my gestures and the intentions discernible in the conduct of other people. It is as if the other person's intentions inhabited my body and mine his.
>
> (Merleau-Ponty, 1962)

The healing that unfolds is beyond what can unfold in the analytic dyad and beyond verbally based group work. The work does not replace the more verbal dialogues of analytical work; it adds to it and furthers it.

Plumbing the depths of intimacy with self in this way can occur because of being relationally felt by others in the circle. The work blossoms into something beyond the analytic third because groups are not a dyad—it gives birth to something beyond the third. This is a group, a conscious collective of others, both human and nonhuman others, giving rise to not simply the analytic third but a relational whole.

Participants' First-person Narratives (continued)

The Last Mover to Speak

After resting on the ground for an extended time, I know I must stand. I kneel first and then push myself to an upright, standing position. My eyes are closed, and I am struck by how high up I am—I feel so far from the ground. I know then that I must not just stand; I must walk. I turn to my left and begin walking. It is so dark. So, so dark. Darker than it has ever been. I cannot see a thing. I am afraid I will bump my head on a beam even though there is not one. I hesitantly walk, fumbling my way in the darkness. I bump into another mover. Huh. I have reached a fork in the road.

Although there is a sense of loss in not engaging with the other mover, I am determined to keep walking. My toes find a familiar seam in the carpet, and I am able to somewhat locate myself. I step over the seam and onwards. It is so dark. I cannot see anything. I feel like Bambi walking, wobbling through the dark. I scan the darkness with my feet and my hands. I find the edge of the carpet, and I bump into a Witness. I am surprised; I did not even think this was an option. I hear the bell ring.

I Witness

I hear you speak of your determination to see this journey through, though you go knowing you are in the utter dark. You speak of concern that you may bump into beams. In my story, I imagine these as old structures imprinted in your body-mind, and now, as you find your way in the dark, you work to release these old imprints and discover new territory.

The sometimes expressive, sometimes imperceptible movements and subtle gestures that arise in the practice fall between everyday actions and dance. The contemplative nature transforms the most pedestrian of gestures into something that witnesses, whose eyes are open, are compelled to attend to and discover what happens next, as they feel to be an intrinsic part of the unfolding. The distinction between witnesses and movers softens as the group's focused attention and affective field heightens. Each is highly affected. Because of the intention for each to maintain a strong inner witness, this softening of boundaries is not based on psychophysical merger. If that were to dominate, a sense of murky deadness would emerge.

The Retreat Comes to a Close

This final mover, who knows she must go on without knowing where her steps will take her, exemplifies Linda Hogan's words on the ceremony's closure, which I read to the group before we part:

> The ceremony is a point of return. It takes us toward a place of balance, our place in the community of all things. It is an event that sets us back upright. But it is not a finished thing. The real ceremony begins where the formal one ends, when we take up a new way, our minds and hearts filled with the vision of earth that holds us within it, in compassionate relationship to and with our world.
>
> (Hogan, 1995, pp. 40–41)

Settling into this inward realm is often felt as a coming home. Mary Whitehouse reminds us, "To get to this authenticity, a sacrifice is involved" (Frantz, 1999/1972, p. 23). We make sacred that which we set aside, sacrificing the pulls and complexities of everyday life—the concrete activities, habitual attitudes, and familiar ego stances—and enter into silence with ourselves and each other.[10] This practice is an invitation to set aside the known, habitual, everyday way we create a boundary impermeable to a more vulnerable inner reality. Throughout history and cultures, through formal observances, exacting procedures, and spontaneous arisings, people have created dances, rituals, and ceremonies. The psychological perspective intrinsic to Movement in Depth brings a contemporary nuance to this ancient impulse. I have facilitated groups in the United States, Brazil, Spain, Japan, China, and Korea. My experience working with people from these cultures is that this non-conceptually based mode of understanding often feels familiar, easy to enter, and closely related to something they have always known. Differences in language become less of a barrier and more of a resource. When working with groups composed of persons from many different cultural backgrounds, I have seen that the practice affords participants more accessible access to their traditional knowledge than more dyadic verbally based therapy. Working with groups such as this has been some of my professional life's most moving and enriching experiences.

The Neuroscientific Basis of Interaffectivity

Microanalysis of the affective life unfolding in groups gives us a window into something significant about our profound mutual influence on one another. What becomes apparent is the extraordinary degree that we are non-consciously influencing and affecting each other all the time. The practice of Movement in Depth becomes a meditation on how each action, thought, and feeling matters. It matters to ourselves and to each other. Through it, we learn how permeable our boundaries are. This is not solely a matter of choice. We are neurologically wired, "an intertwinement of two cycles of embodied affectivity, thus continuously modifying each partner's affective affordances and bodily resonance" (Fuchs & Koch, 2014, p. 1). In a circular and reciprocal cycle, we become resonant and responsive to the other's affective states. With this awareness, we can choose how we relate to what arises and consciously navigate our effect on and openness to each other.

Cultural and developmental processes lay the groundwork for either mutuality and reciprocation or more rigid boundaried postures of our sense of self in relation to the other. In cultures with a high value on individuality and autonomy, there are times when individuals and groups exploring this practice discover an embodied attitudinal softening and a new experience of what is possible in relationships. Alternately, in cultures emphasizing being one within the greater collective, participants, not infrequently, discover a felt possibility of differentiation and individual freedom.

What unfolds within the resonant field of this practice often feels mysterious and engenders an experience of the numinous in participants. This resonant field has been referred to as intercorporeality by phenomenologists, and the intersubjective field by psychologists. Infant research coupled with neuroscience has given rise to the term interaffectivity, bridging these diverse fields of study. Perhaps most mysterious is the unknown potential of what is possible when we bring intention to cultivate an attuned, caring, psychologically informed, non-judgmental attitude toward ourselves and each other in groups. We do not know the limits of this. Just as is oppositely true—there seems to be no known bound to how cruel we can be to each other, whether consciously or unconsciously intended. While Jung and others abhor the unconscious trance of the "collective" and spoke of the necessity to differentiate from it, we have yet to consciously cultivate what is possible when we gather, collaborate, and create in an atmosphere of psychologically informed relating. If conscious intent is not cultivated in our interactions, our neurological wiring operates outside of our awareness, and we affect and act toward each other based on interaffective resonance, for better or for ill.

The Crucial Function of Making Shadow Material Conscious

It might seem that I am speaking of work with individuals or groups devoid of conflict, animosity, and other complicated feelings. However, our thoughts, feelings, and actions need not be stripped of shadow in such a practice. On the contrary, the shadow must be made conscious and reflected on, so choice is made conscious. If disavowed, a deadness or unresolvable tension arises in the group dynamic. If we attempt to strip ourselves of the shadow elements rather than reflect and work with them as they arise, we erase the vital forces that move through us. Jung referred to holding the tension of the opposites within and struggling with that tension rather than splitting or dissociating as the transcendent function. It is through the conscious holding that a third thing arises, which carries a potential, a new attitude that transcends the either/or split. This is foundational to an inner democracy of self and outer democracy of the collective body (Kalsched, 2023). Seeing through this inner struggle gives rise to the capacity to refrain from projecting it—onto ourselves or each other. This is essential because "when an inner situation is not made conscious, it happens outside, as fate" (Jung, 1951, para. 126).

Vulnerability as Strength

Speaking of her time learning from Mary Whitehouse, Janet Adler recounts:

> To me, she was a strong woman, a strength, that I trusted because I experienced her vulnerability. She knew how, to safely enough, invite those of us who came to work with her, toward opening to our own vulnerability—the source of our own developing strength.
>
> (2022, p. 250)

A dear colleague, the late Neela Haze,[11] revealed one evening to a group to which she was presenting that *"through this practice, my heart opened."* Reflecting on both of these women's words, I can say, through this practice my heart opened beyond what I imagined possible as I learned what was shareable—my most vulnerable wounded places as well as that which I experience as most sacred. I had at one time thought of that realm as an utterly private domain, one I could not communicate to another, in part because of the depths of the nonverbal dimension of my experience of the numinous. What I discovered was how much larger it and I became in communion with others.

Notes

1 This paper was published in Pallaro (Ed.) (1999).
2 Marie-Louise von Franz emphasizes that the compensatory function of the psyche brings balance to the one-sided perspective that our egos tend to adopt, which always feels to be a surprise.
3 The BCSPG, when speaking of something other than interpretation, refers to the level of intersubjective regulation in the domain of implicit knowledge at the local level. The local level refers to the microanalysis of moment-to-moment activity occurring within each individual and between the dyad. This moment-to-moment activity is largely oriented to bodily-based experiencing in relationships that typically occur outside of awareness.
4 Mary Whitehouse considered her work an "approach" rather than a method and referred to it in various ways, including: "Movement in Depth," "The Moving Imagination," and "Authentic Movement." Janet Adler adopted the name Authentic Movement. Adler contributed greatly to the practice, including carefully crafting a structure for group work that provides the emotional safety necessary for the kind of profound exploration possible in the work. Largely based on her contributions, the international community has adopted the name Authentic Movement. I struggle with that naming because the word "authentic" so easily stirs a polarization with "inauthentic." I prefer the name Moving in Depth.
5 This is the first time we have been able to meet indoors in person for three years due to COVID-19. Of the 13 who planned to attend, one could not because she contracted COVID-19 two days before our start.
6 Alton Wasson, co-founder of Contemplative Dance, taught me this simple yet profound practice of moving and being in the greater natural world.
7 See Chapter 4 on bodily-based nonverbal communication between caregiver and child.
8 The eucalyptus tree, whose original habitat is Australia, is a very abundant, beautiful, invasive species in this ecosystem, often sighted for fueling destructive wildfires. Because of this, they hold a paradoxical beauty for those who live here.
9 Later in a letter to the group, when this mover has had time to let words arise, she tells us that the gesture was that of the Buddhist Ksitigarbha Bodhisattva. In Korea, Ksitigarbha is typically represented as gender-neutral or feminine. The feminine form, she likens to Demeter—but in reverse, as in this myth, the daughter goes into the underworld to save her mother.
10 The word "sacrifice" derives from the Latin *sacrificium*, which combines the words *sacer*, meaning something set apart from the secular or profane, holy; and *facere*, meaning to make.
11 Neela Haze and Tina Stromsted founded the Authentic Movement Institute of California. They taught and trained others in Authentic Movement from 1993 to 2004. Both Joan Chodorow and Janet Adler were faculty.

References

Adler, J. (1999/1987). Who is the witness? In P. Pallaro (Ed.), *Authentic movement: Essays by Mary Starks Whitehouse, Janet Adler and Joan Chodorow* (pp. 141–159). London: Jessica Kingsley.

—— (1999/1972). Integrity of body and psyche: Some notes on work in process. In P. Pallaro (Ed.), *Authentic movement: Essays by Mary Starks Whitehouse, Janet Adler and Joan Chodorow*. London: Jessica Kingsley.

—— (1999/1976). Authentic movement and sexuality in the therapeutic experience. In P. Pallaro (Ed.), *Essays by Mary Starks Whitehouse, Janet Adler and Joan Chodorow.* London: Jessica Kingsley.

—— (2002). *Offering from the conscious body: The discipline of authentic movement.* Rochester, VT: Inner Traditions.

Adler, J., Morrissey, B., & Sager, P. (2022). *Intimacy in emptiness: An evolution of embodied consciousness.* Rochester, VT: Inner Traditions.

Boston Change Process Study Group (BCPSG). (2018). Moving through and being moved by: embodiment in development and in the therapeutic relationship. *Contemporary Psychoanalysis, 54*(2), 299–321. https://doi.org/10.1080/00107530.2018.1456841

Castle, J. (2001). When the floor is the couch: The use of movement in depth psychotherapy, presented January 11, 2001, at the Northwest Alliance for Psychoanalytic Study.

Chodorow, J. (1999/1986). The body as symbol: Dance/movement in analysis. In P. Pallaro (Ed.), *Authentic movement: Essays by Mary Starks Whitehouse, Janet Adler and Joan Chodorow.* London: Jessica Kingsley.

——(1999/1977). Dance therapy and the transcendent function. In P. Pallaro (Ed.), *Essays by Mary Starks Whitehouse, Janet Adler and Joan Chodorow.* London: Jessica Kingsley.

——(1999/1984). To move and be moved. In P. Pallaro (Ed.), *Essays by Mary Starks Whitehouse, Janet Adler and Joan Chodorow.* London: Jessica Kingsley.

—— (1991). *Dance therapy and depth psychology: The moving imagination.* London: Routledge.

Fleischer, K. (2023). Collective trauma, implicit memories, the body, and active imagination in Jungian analysis. *Journal of Analytical Psychology, 68*(2), 395–415. https://doi.org/10.1111/1468-5922.12908

Frantz, G. (1999/1972). An approach to the center: An interview with Mary Whitehouse. In P. Pallaro (Ed.), *Essays by Mary Starks Whitehouse, Janet Adler and Joan Chodorow.* London: Jessica Kingsley

Fuchs, T. (2017). Intercorporeality and interaffectivity. In C. Meyer, J. Streeck, & J. S. Jordan (Eds.), *Intercorporeality: Emerging socialities in interaction.* Oxford: Oxford University Press. https://doi.org/10.1093/acprof:oso/9780190210465.003.0001

—— (2020). Embodied interaffectivity and psychopathology. In H. L. Maibom (Ed.), *The Routledge handbook of phenomenology of emotion* (pp. 28–40). London, New York: Routledge. https://doi.org/10.4324/9781315180786-31

Fuchs, T., & Koch S. C. (2014). Embodied affectivity: On moving and being moved. *Frontiers in Psychology, 5.* https://doi.org/10.3389/fpsyg.2014.00508

Gendlin, E.T. (1962). *Experiencing and the creation of meaning: A philosophical and psychological approach to the subjective.* Glencoe, IL: Free Press.

—— (1995). Crossing and dipping: Some terms for approaching the interface between natural understanding and logical formulation. *Minds and Machines: Journal for Artificial Intelligence, Philosophy and Cognitive Science, 5*(4), 547–560. https://doi.org/10.1007/BF00974985

—— (1997). *A process model: Studies in phenomenology and existential philosophy.* New York: The International Focusing Institute.

—— (2017). *Saying what we mean: Implicit precision and the responsive order.* Evanston, IL: Northwestern University Press.

Hogan, L. (1995). *Dwellings: A spiritual history of the living world.* New York: W. W. Norton.

Holifield, B. (2007). Against the wall her beating heart: Somatic dimensions of transference and countertransference. In P. Pallaro (Ed.), *Authentic movement: Moving the body, moving the self, being moved: A collection of essays, vol. 2*. London: Jessica Kingsley.

Jung, C. G. (1951). Aion: Researches into the phenomenology of the self. In *The collected works of C. G. Jung, vol. 9ii*, R. F. C. Hull (Trans.). Princeton, NJ: Princeton University Press.

—— (1972/1954). On the nature of the psyche. In *The collected works of C. G. Jung, vol. 8*, 2nd ed. Princeton, NJ: Princeton University Press.

Kalsched, D. (2023). Inner and outer democracy and the threat of authoritarianism, "with Ukrainian Jungians." Webinar # 8 September 19, 2023, Archive for Research in Archetypal Symbolism, webinars from the #WithUkranianJungians project. https://aras.org/wujwebinars.

Merleau-Ponty, M. (1962). *The phenomenology of perception*. New York: Humanities Press.

Musicant, S. (2007). Authentic movement in clinical work. In P. Pallaro (Ed.), *Authentic movement: Moving the body, moving the self, being moved: A collection of essays, vol. 2*. London: Jessica Kingsley.

Pallaro, P. (Ed.). (1999). *Authentic movement: Essays by Mary Starks Whitehouse, Janet Adler and Joan Chodorow*. London: Jessica Kingsley.

—— (Ed.). (2007). *Authentic movement: Moving the body, moving the self, being moved: A collection of essays*. London: Jessica Kingsley.

—— (2007). Somatic transference: The therapist in relationship. In P. Pallaro (Ed.), *Authentic movement: Moving the body, moving the self, being moved: A collection of essays, vol. 2*. London: Jessica Kingsley.

Stromsted, T. (2007). The dancing body in psychotherapy. In P. Pallaro (Ed.), *Authentic movement: Moving the body, moving the self, being moved: A collection of essays, vol. 2*. London: Jessica Kingsley.

Wasson, A. (2007). Witnessing and the chest of drawers. In P. Pallaro (Ed.), *Authentic movement: Moving the body, moving the self, being moved: A collection of essays, vol. 2*. London: Jessica Kingsley.

Watkins, M. (2022). Individuation, ancestral reckoning, and ecopsychosocial repair. Psychosocial Wednesdays on YouTube: www.youtube.com/watch?v=iS0QTbS--uY

Whitehouse, M. S. (1999/1956). Creative expression in physical movement is language without words.In P. Pallaro (Ed.), *Essays by Mary Starks Whitehouse, Janet Adler and Joan Chodorow*. London: Jessica Kingsley.

—— (1999/1995). The Tao of the body. In P. Pallaro (Ed.), *Essays by Mary Starks Whitehouse, Janet Adler and Joan Chodorow*. London: Jessica Kingsley.

—— (1999/1987). Physical movement and personality. In P. Pallaro (Ed.), *Essays by Mary Starks Whitehouse, Janet Adler and Joan Chodorow*. London: Jessica Kingsley.

—— (1999/1977). The transference and dance therapy. In P. Pallaro (Ed.), *Essays by Mary Starks Whitehouse, Janet Adler and Joan Chodorow*. London: Jessica Kingsley

—— (1999/1979). C. G. Jung and dance therapy: Two major priciples. In P. Pallaro (Ed.), *Essays by Mary Starks Whitehouse, Janet Adler and Joan Chodorow*. London: Jessica Kingsley.

Wyman-McGinty, W. (2007). The body in analysis: Authentic movement and witnessing in analytic practice. In P. Pallaro (Ed.), *Authentic movement: Moving the body, moving the self, being moved: A collection of essays, vol. 2*. London: Jessica Kingsley.

Conclusion

I developed this book based on a non-dualistic perspective because I wished to reach beyond the categorical tendencies that draw distinctions between psyche and body, observer and observed, therapist and patient, humans and the natural world, spirit and matter.

While I challenge those polarities, it is clear we often *feel* these categorical distinctions as our existential or psychic reality. The feeling of being separate from and fragmented within the living medium of one's own bodied nature is not new, having arisen across time and culture. This opens questions of why and how this is so, and beckons inquiry into how we might find a way through these feelings and perceptions. What is the "way in" to another possibility?

I have explored this inquiry from the perspective of cultural influences, affective neuroscience, and infant development. Additionally, I have included exploration of the psychophysical experience of working with trauma in a somatically informed depth psychotherapeutic approach. It is my hope that this broadens and deepens the work by addressing the question of why and how it is that, at times, we feel disconnected from our bodies, our emotions and a sense of the numinosity of lived experience. The inwardly felt body, when engaged with curiosity in the company of a responsive therapist, reveals a more nuanced feel of lived experience, reconnecting those broken links. While this is of great importance when trauma has severed the link to one's body and emotional life, it is of equal importance in cultivating the dimensional life one longs for.

Somatically informed depth psychotherapeutic processes that work to heal trauma have shown how, when healing[1] does occur, a transformation process is often set in motion that awakens a sense of profound integration of these polarities. This unfolds as layers of implicit processes that have occurred at interoceptive, pre-affective, pre-reflective, affective, and imagistic levels are brought to awareness and processed within a therapeutic relationship. When one *directly experiences* the underlying unity of body and psyche, spirit and matter, nature and self, or deep interconnectedness with another, it often gives way to a sublime sense of wonder, of being part of something bigger than oneself.

A non-dualistic perspective emphasizes direct experiential knowing while holding the value of conceptual and scientific understandings. Reaching back at least as

DOI: 10.4324/9781003305804-11

far as the Enlightenment period, abstract forms of knowledge that privilege spirit over matter have held favor over those that are sensorial, kinesthetic, or affective. The primacy of bodily-based knowing revealed through infant research illuminates an interior world of sensorial apprehension that conceptually based knowing and psychoanalytic thought often overlook. Furthermore, it establishes the body as intrinsic to relational life. Freud's 1923 statement that "The ego is first and foremost a bodily ego," is as cogent today as it was then (1961, p. 26). It has only been confirmed by infant research and affective neuroscience. Psychic life is born in the body and is sustained by the body. It is in and through the body that relationship begins. Disruptions in one's earliest relationship with the primary caregiver are synonymous with disruption of the integral unity of psyche and body.

Affective neuroscience reveals the emergence of consciousness intrinsically rooted in bodily life (Fuchs, 2018; Damasio, 2021). It also illuminates the intricate sensory-motor and neurological basis of affects. Moreover, neuroscience has established the anatomical-functional foundations of intersubjective life. Interaffectivity, a term D. N. Stern (2018/1985, p. 132) uses to describe the affective resonance that unfolds between parents and infants, was extended by Fuchs (2017) to convey the reciprocal and circular neural basis of mutual influence between persons—what Gallese refers to as "we-centric space" (2012). According to Gallese, who along with a team of others, discovered mirror neurons, "we-ness and intersubjectivity ontologically ground the human condition, in which reciprocity foundationally defines human existence" (2012, p. 62). These findings illuminate what we sometimes know we feel but which are hard to express conceptually. I find these insights that have emerged from neuroscience and infant research enhance both my thinking about and experiential feel of embodied subjectivity and intersubjective experience.

Reflections on Dyadic Work

The vignettes and case studies I have presented offer a window into both the analysand's and my experience of the somatic dimension of psychic life in a depth psychotherapeutic process that incorporates the body. Through these examples, I have sought to provide a vivid and detailed description of my interactions with clients, highlighting the ways in which the work influences my own psyche-somatic process.

I highlight the organizing role that felt sensation, sensory perception, and affective experience have on facilitating the re-establishment of psyche indwelling the soma. Because disruptions of the felt sense of psyche integral to soma occur in infancy, work of this nature falls out of the purview of traditional psychoanalysis. "It requires instead a working-through focused on the present, on the heart of the analytic relationship, and on the activation of an awareness of one's own inner mode of functioning" (Lombardi, 2017, p. 23). Focus on direct sensorial and relational experience in the body is foundational in working with the analysand's unformulated experience. As this occurs, affects are able to be borne, reflected on, and lived as feelings-in-the-body while simultaneously making way for the establishment of new relational organizations. Throughout the clinical examples, I have shown how the mythopoetic imagination and soma entwine—at times, attention to the somatic dimension stirs the creative unconscious in the form of dreams, active imagination, artworks, and movement. Reciprocally, the imaginal world informs and stimulates somatic experience. In this way, the mythopoetic reality revealed in a depth analysis weaves somatic experience into a tapestry of personal meaning, facilitating deep psychophysical transformation. The body is both a portal to and the medium of experiencing the numinous dimensions of the soul's life—to healing and wholeness that goes far beyond just the relief of traumatic symptoms, leading to an increased access to feelings in general and to a renewed sense of soulful aliveness.

By bringing these aspects of therapeutic work together, I hope to have offered a deeper understanding of the complex interplay of psyche and body and to demonstrate the profound importance of bringing the body into the practice of depth psychotherapy for healing trauma *and* enhancing daily life.

Interaffectivity in Authentic Movement Group Practice

In Chapter 9, using all of these threads of relational understanding as a backdrop, I delve deeper into interaffectivity as experienced among group members in the work of Authentic Movement. Whether done as group psychotherapy or as contemplative practice, this approach serves as a portal or "way in" to what I call the poetics of embodiment.

In that chapter, I have made room for the detailed narrative that arose in one particular retreat. A vivid description of direct experience offers a way into the intimacy of moment-to-moment unfolding, and this is what being in the body is about—being in the rich nuance of unfolding felt experience.

In daily discourse, in the context of a Western cultural mode of relating, we typically move to a more conceptual form of description in which we talk about what happened, using interpretive formulations that offer an integrative overview of an event. The overview, which usually offers shortcuts to the telling of an experience, though useful, is a top-down mode of expression. By this, I mean talking about experience from a more conceptually centered perspective.

In its detailed and careful attention to felt experience unfolding in time, the experience-near approach, which is a more bottom-up mode of expression, one speaks from the experience rather than about it. Illuminating interaffectivity via the medium of the experienced body reveals the unfolding nuance of intimacy with self, other, and the world occurs at a different tempo than conceptually driven modes of relationship. Perhaps analogous to the left and right hand playing piano— though synchronized, the specific tempo or speed of each may vary. There is a great loss if playing is constrained to just one hand. Such constraints imposed on relational domains create a negative feedback loop. The more that concepts dominate our expression, the more distant we become from direct experience. The more distanced from direct experience, the more our perceptions become dominated by concept and objectification rather than subjective experience. Caught in that negative feedback loop, we run the risk of eclipsing of the body (Ferrari, 2004)—of losing track of felt experience. "The body," says Gallese, "is the main source of meaning, because it not only structures the experiential aspects of interpersonal relations, but also their linguistic representations" (2009, p. 533).

Neuroscience That Highlights Unity of Body and Mind

The perspective forwarded by affective neuroscience that consciousness co-arises with bodily life challenges typical Western thought that suggests consciousness infuses the body from a hierarchically situated source. This basic *feeling* of being alive and its affective affordances are further elaborated as interoception of the deep body meets exteroception of the outer world, which, within microseconds, is processed in the cortical regions of our embodied brain, giving rise to affects. Affects are in the body and could not be otherwise. From an affective neuroscientific perspective, we are embodied beings. As I have reviewed in Chapter 2, the *awareness* of these interoceptive and exteroceptive states gives rise to *a felt sense* of affects, embodiment, and affect tolerance. This felt sense of embodiment can be cultivated. Engaging the body inevitably engages the somatic unconscious. Bringing skilled attention to the body in depth psychotherapy furthers the endeavor of a felt sense of embodiment, simultaneously bridging the relationship between the conscious and unconscious. This deepens the dimensionality of our work with affect, trauma, and transformative energies of the numinous.

Biological Factors That Contribute to the Feeling of Separation of Psyche and Body

Though there are cultural, developmental, and trauma-related factors that contribute to a felt sense of body separate from psyche, there are also biological factors that do so as well. While there are realms of the body we can subjectively experience, there are also realms that most of us do not have access to—what could be called the objective body[2] (Fuchs, 2020). Examples of this are physiological processes such as those of the spleen, pancreas, liver, and gallbladder. Here lies an experiential basis of "one's" body as separate from "one's self," that is, one's subjective experience of self. Additionally, the entire body can be referred to in the third person as an object—by self or another. Regardless of our personal or cultural context, each of us typically has some subjective experience of our body and an absence of felt awareness of the inaccessible aspects of the body.

The Jungian perspective of cultivating a relationship with one's inner life includes doing so with that aspect of the Self that is unknowable. The Self represents the totality of the person, including an unknowable essence that exceeds our comprehension, indicating its divine and mysterious nature.

I will end here with the dilemma we encounter between the bodily basis of our sense of subjective self and that which lies beyond experiential knowing. Throughout this book, I have explored multiple "ways in" to developing relationships with our own-bodied self and others' personed bodies.

However, our bodies will always present us with what is beyond our knowing and in which we have little or no say. While we can cultivate conditions and work on hoped-for outcomes within, we will always face that which is beyond our ultimate control. Life and death are the penultimate aspects of this reality; a mystery (*mysterium*) that can be at once terrifying (*tremendum*) and fascinating (*fascinans*) thus arousing a sense of the numinous (Otto, 1923). The same could be said about relating to the other—we can listen, attune with, and accompany, yet aspects of the other will always remain unknowable. Moreover, what happens between us ultimately contains something beyond our capacity to fully know.

The Body a Facet of the Mysterium Coniunctionis

It is in relating to that unknown within myself, as lived in my body, that I experience another facet of Jung's concept of the *Mysterium Coniunctionis*—the paradoxical mystery of the union of the opposites (1970/1963). Grappling with this ever-present inner mystery is one of the great tasks of a lifetime—of individuation. Perhaps because of this tension between the subjectively experienced body and the objective unknowable body, there will inevitably be a fluctuating spectrum of an integral unity of psyche/self and body and a gap between psyche/self and body.

The South Asian feminine deity, Akhilandeshwari—she who is never not broken—comes to my awareness here. In Shakta Tantra, a tradition in Hinduism that views the godhead metaphorically as nature such that the microcosm is the macrocosm, Akhilandeshwari is broken because we and the world are broken. She is a powerful force in the cosmic field of consciousness. It is through our awareness of brokenness—fragmentation/gaps—that light gets in. The light is our awareness, our consciousness. As we bring awareness to the fragmentation, paradoxically, we are re-made whole, again and again (Amazzone, 2015).

Notes

1 By healing here, I mean the feeling of being whole in oneself or on a path toward a wholeness that may be a worthy endeavor that one never fully attains—such as Jung's Individuation or the alchemist's "The Great Work."
2 Fuchs (2020) describes this as the body–body problem rather than a mind–body problem.

References

Amazzone, L. (2015). Akhilandeshwari: The power of brokenness. *Sutra Journal: Eternal Truths, Modern Voices*. www.sutrajournal.com/akhilandeshwari-the-power-of-brokenness-by-laura-amazzone

Damasio, A. (2021). *Feeling and knowing: Making minds conscious*. New York: Pantheon Books.

Ferrari, A. B. (2004). *From the eclipse of the body to the dawn of thought*. London: Free Association Books.

Freud, S. (1961). *The ego and the id*. New York: W. W. Norton.

Fuchs, T. (2017). Intercorporeality and interaffectivity. In C. Meyer, J. Streeck, & J. S. Jordan (Eds.), *Intercorporeality: Emerging socialities in interaction, foundations of human interaction*. New York: Oxford University Press. https://doi.org/10.1093/acprof: oso/9780190210465.003.0001

——— (2018). *Ecology of the brain*. Oxford: Oxford University Press.

——— (2020). The circularity of the embodied mind. *Frontiers in Psychology 11*. https:// doi.org/10.3389/fpsyg.2020.01707

Gallese, V. (2009). Mirror neurons, embodied simulation, and the neural basis of social identification. *Psychoanalytic Dialogues*, *19*(5), 519–536.

——— (2012). Embodied simulation theory and intersubjectivity. Mulino: Corisco Edizioni. www.coriscoedizioni.it/wp-content/uploads/2012/11/Gallese-Embodied-Simulation-Theory.pdf

Jung, C. G. (1970/1963). *Mysterium coniunctionis: An inquiry into the separation and synthesis of psychic opposites in alchemy*. R. F. C. Hull (Trans.). In H. Read, M. Fordham, & G. Adler (Eds.), *The collected works of C. G. Jung: vol. 9*. Princeton, NJ: Princeton University Press.

Lombardi, R. (2017). *Body–mind dissociation in psychoanalysis: Development after Bion*. (Relational Perspective Book Series). (Kindle edition) London, New York: Routledge.

Otto, R. (1923). *The idea of the holy*. Oxford: Oxford University Press.

Stern, D. N. (2018/1985). *The interpersonal world of the infant*. New York: Basic Books.

Index